European School of Oncology

# Monographs

Series Editor: U. Veronesi

A. Goldhirsch (Ed.)

# Endocrine Therapy of Breast Cancer IV

With 19 Figures and 40 Tables

Springer-Verlag Berlin Heidelberg New York
London Paris Tokyo Hong Kong Barcelona

A. Goldhirsch

Department of Medical Oncology
Ospedale Civico
via Tesserete 46
6900 Lugano, Switzerland

The European School of Oncology gratefully acknowledges sponsorship for the Task Force received from

ICI **Pharmaceuticals**

Library of Congress Cataloging-in-Publication Data
Endocrine therapy of breast cancer IV / A. Goldhirsch (ed.). p. cm.–(Monographs European School of Oncology)
ISBN-13: 978-3-642-75950-5 e-ISBN-13: 978-3-642-75948-2
DOI: 10.1007/ 978-3-642-75948-2
1. Breast–Cancer–Hormone therapy. I. Goldhirsch, A. (Aron)
II. Series. III. Series: Monographs (European School of Oncology) RC280.B8E523 1990 616.99'449061–dc20 DNLM/DLC
for Library of Congress 90-10158 CIP


Softcover reprint of the hardcover 1st edition 1990



2123/3145-543210 – Printed on acid-free paper

# Foreword

The European School of Oncology came into existence to respond to a need for information, education and training in the field of the diagnosis and treatment of cancer. There are two main reasons why such an initiative was considered necessary. Firstly, the teaching of oncology requires a rigorously multidisciplinary approach which is difficult for the Universities to put into practice since their system is mainly disciplinary orientated. Secondly, the rate of technological development that impinges on the diagnosis and treatment of cancer has been so rapid that it is not an easy task for medical faculties to adapt their curricula flexibly.

With its residential courses for organ pathologies and the seminars on new techniques (laser, monoclonal antibodies, imaging techniques etc.) or on the principal therapeutic controversies (conservative or mutilating surgery, primary or adjuvant chemotherapy, radiotherapy alone or integrated), it is the ambition of the European School of Oncology to fill a cultural and scientific gap and, thereby, create a bridge between the University and Industry and between these two and daily medical practice.

One of the more recent initiatives of ESO has been the institution of permanent study groups, also called task forces, where a limited number of leading experts are invited to meet once a year with the aim of defining the state of the art and possibly reaching a consensus on future developments in specific fields of oncology.

The ESO Monograph series was designed with the specific purpose of disseminating the results of these study group meetings, and providing concise and updated reviews of the topic discussed.

It was decided to keep the layout relatively simple, in order to restrict the costs and make the monographs available in the shortest possible time, thus overcoming a common problem in medical literature: that of the material being outdated even before publication.

UMBERTO VERONESI
Chairman Scientific Committee
European School of Oncology

# Contents

# Introduction

A. Goldhirsch

Division of Oncology, Ospedale San Giovanni, Bellinzona, and Ospedale Civico, Lugano, Switzerland

This is the fourth issue of our Monograph on Endocrine Therapy of Breast Cancer. As in the past, this volume is the result of highly interesting discussions among the members of the Task Force and several guests, all of them outstanding researchers in their respective fields. To discuss controversial issues pertaining to data deriving from one's own work is an extremely pleasant exercise, and at the same time generates both sound criticism and new hypotheses; the latter is essential for the continuation of productive research. The 1990 edition contains the following four items of notable interest: 1) new data concerning the function of oestrogen and progesterone in promoting receptor-mediated growth; 2) a definition of prognostic factors in breast cancer, particularly in node-negative disease; 3) new data about "old" endocrine therapies; and 4) a discussion of adjuvant therapies and the measure of their benefit, with special emphasis on quality-of-life considerations.

Each of the chapters provides new data or discusses features of interest to individuals who are intellectually involved with breast cancer: Dr. King challenges the role of oestrogens in cell growth and differentiation by introducing new "actors", progesterone and progestins. New views regarding receptors and oestrogen are discussed by Dr. Milgrom. The prognosis of breast cancer is reviewed by Dr. Klijn, especially in relation to growth factors and their receptors, and by Dr. Mouridsen and other members of the Danish Breast Cancer Study Group, who report their findings about node-negative disease. In a section on endocrine therapeutics, Dr. Jordan provides new data on the long-term use of tamoxifen, Dr. Howell discusses endocrine mechanisms which should be reconsidered and re-examined, and Dr. Milsted reviews the status of LHRH-superanalogues. Adjuvant systemic therapies are also dealt with by Dr. Kaufmann in his review of new node-negative trials, and by Drs. Gelber, Castiglione and Goldhirsch, whose new data indicate that endocrine mechanisms are not solely responsible for the effect of adjuvant systemic chemotherapy in premenopausal patients. The methodological controversy about how best to define the benefit from a therapy which provides only modest treatment effects is extensively described by Dr. Gelber.

Endocrine mechanisms and breast cancer continue to be fascinating subjects for research which represent fertile areas for the germination of hypotheses. When the Task Force will meet and produce its fifth edition in 1991, new revelations are certain to have come to light which will serve both to nurture and reward our interest in this field.

# Role of Oestrogen and Progestin in Human Mammary Carcinogenesis

R. J. B. King

Imperial Cancer Research Fund Breast Biology Group, Biochemistry Department, University of Surrey, Guildford, Surrey GU2 5XH, United Kingdom

From an endocrinological aspect, the view that oestrogens are the major adverse factor in human breast cancer has dominated thinking in this area [1,2]. This opinion is based on three main lines of evidence; (a) the ability of oestrogens to generate mammary tumours in rodents [3,4]; (b) epidemiologically-derived risk factors such as the protective effect of ovariectomy and increased risk of breast cancer in young women given diethylstilboestrol to prevent abortion [1,2]; and (c) the mitogenic effects of oestrogens on established breast cancer cell lines [5,6] and efficacy of antioestrogens in treating established breast cancer [7].

Conversely, the other ovarian steroid progesterone and its synthetic derivatives (progestins) are thought to be protective, a view largely based on their antioestrogenic and therefore antiproliferative effects on endometrium [8]. Supportive evidence for beneficial effects of progestins comes from their clinical use in advanced breast cancer [9] and their ability to decrease tumour yield under certain conditions in rodents [3,4].

Many of the data on which the above model is based are capable of the alternative explanation that, as far as early stages of breast cancer induction are concerned, progestins are not good but bad and oestrogens may play a more permissive role. This has been termed the "oestrogen plus progestagen" hypothesis [10], which is mainly based on two types of observations. In contrast to endometrium, *in vivo* proliferation of normal human breast epithelium is maximal during the progestagenic phase of the cycle and the contraceptive pill stimulates proliferation [11-15] together with publications suggesting an increased risk of breast cancer in young women on the contraceptive pill [16,17] and with one report of a progestin-related breast cancer risk in women on hormone replacement therapy [18]. It must, however, be stressed that neither of these sets of epidemiological data should be considered proven.

Given the importance of deciding whether oestrogen alone or oestrogen plus progestin adversely affects human breast cancer, resolution of the question is imperative. Currently, insufficient data are available to achieve this objective. The purpose of this chapter is to highlight some of the more important points that need resolution.

## Animal Studies

Oestrogens alone can induce mammary tumours in mice [3,4]; this could be used as evidence against a progestin involvement. However, a progestagenic environment increases tumour incidence [3,4], so progestins can be stimulatory. The endocrine requirements of hydrocarbon-induced mammary tumours are complex and vary according to species and whether the manipulations are carried out before or after hydrocarbon administration. Depending on conditions, progestins can either decrease or increase tumour development [3,4,19]. Thus, in relation to the human situation, the animal data are inconclusive in deciding between the two models.

## Risk Factors

Ovariectomy clearly protects against subsequent development of breast cancer [1,2] but, as this operation removes both oestrogen and progestin, its interpretation is equivocal. Likewise, increased tumour incidence in women who received diethylstilboestrol for threatened abortion occurred against the progestagenic background of pregnancy [1,2]; increased progestin potency in that oestrogenic environment cannot be discounted. The increased risk due to obesity [1,2] could be explained in the same way for premenopausal women, but the postmenopausal situation would be more problematic.

In the original "bad oestrogen" hypothesis, it was thought that, with early menarche, the initial cycles were anovulatory and therefore progestin deficient [20], but this is now thought to be incorrect [21,22], so that early menarche establishes early exposure to progesterone. Thus, the "oestrogen alone" model is less compatible with the menarche data than the "oestrogen plus progestin" hypothesis.

Late menopause [1,2] does not immediately fit with the progestin model as such cycles tend to be anovular [22]; several explanations are possible. If hormonal sensitivity changes with progression (see below), it is possible that the breast cells at risk are different at the two extremes of reproductive life and that they should be considered as being at different stages of progression. Alternatively, one could argue, as others have done [22], that the total number of ovulatory cycles (oestrogen and progestin) is the important feature and that the late menopause reflects an increased number of such cycles, even though the last ones are anovular.

An early, first full-term pregnancy markedly decreases the risk of subsequent breast cancer, an effect that has been ascribed to the highly progestagenic milieu of pregnancy [1,2]. This could argue against a bad effect of progestins, but the hormonal environment of pregnancy is not the same as that of the luteal phase and this is reflected in the physiological response of the mammary lobules. In the normal cycle, the intense lobular development associated with pregnancy does not occur and epithelial dedifferentiation is less evident [19]. Pregnancy-related differentiation makes the epithelial cells more resistant to carcinogens [19], an effect that may not occur in the normal cycle. Intriguingly, pregnancy results in a long-term desensitisation to the proliferating effects of the contraceptive pill on breast epithelium [12].

Explaining the various risk factors by either model alone is difficult. More biological data are required about the various physiological situations that can be related to the rather heterogeneous collection of risk factors.

## Mitogenic Effects of Oestrogens; Antioestrogenic Effects of Progestins

Cell proliferation is a vital component in carcinogenesis both at the level of increasing the number of target cells for initiating agents and in amplifying abnormal cell populations after initiation. Hence, oestrogen and progestin effects on proliferation are relevant to the topic of this chapter.

Most of the data on female sex steroids and cell proliferation have been generated from studies on normal endometrium and breast cancer cell lines. As there is a possibility that hormone sensitivity alters during progression (see below), effects on normal and cancer cells will be considered separately.

### *Normal Cells*

There is no doubt that oestrogens are mitogens for endometrial cells and that progestins counteract that effect [8], but the relevance of those data to normal human breast epithelium is questionable. Several groups have demonstrated that normal breast lobular-alveolar epithelium exhibits greater proliferation in the luteal than follicular phase of the menstrual cycle [11-15]. This clear-cut difference to endometrium indicates that, if oestrogens stimulate breast epithelial proliferation, it is by a less direct route than with endometrium and progestins could be a component distal to oestrogen in the breast. The simplest explanation of the *in vivo* breast data is that progesterone is the proliferative agent, a view that is enhanced by the finding that the contraceptive pill, in particular progestin-only pills, increases luteal phase proliferation [12]. At the very least, there are no data that progestins inhibit oestrogen-induced proliferation in normal, human breast epithelium *in vivo*. In cell culture the situation may be different (see below).

A proliferative effect of progestins could result either in an increased number of targets for initiating agents or change the susceptibility of the epithelial cells to those agents.

Oestrogens, by increasing progesterone receptor levels, are known to increase progestin potency. This could also occur with human mammary epithelium. Alternatively, oestrogens might have a direct mitogenic effect other than via progesterone receptor, although the *in vivo* data indicate that, if so, the effect is small in relation to that of progestins. There is a very low proliferation during the oestrogenic phase of the cycle [11-15], which could be due either to a basal activity or an oestrogenic influence. These *in vivo* data are at variance with cell-culture [23] and nude-mouse [24] results indicating that oestrogens are mitogenic for human mammary epithelium and progestins are inhibitory. The basis for these discrepant results should be urgently identified. Four independent groups have established that, *in vivo*, lobular epithelium proliferates faster during the luteal phase of the cycle [11-15], so this can be taken as proven. An indirect effect of progestins on mammary epithelium is one possible explanation of the discrepant behaviour in culture and *in vivo*, but would not explain the nude-mouse data without invoking species differences. This is an unlikely explanation as rodent mammary epithelium behaves like the human in proliferating out of phase with that of uterine epithelium [25].

### Established Breast Cancer

Oestrogens are well established as being the main steroidal mitogens for established breast cancer [5-7] and may well promote preneoplastic lesions to a more malignant state. Given the menstrual cycle and pill data indicating a proliferative effect of progestins on normal epithelium (see above), it is possible that a change in sensitivity profile occurs at some state in the carcinogenic process.

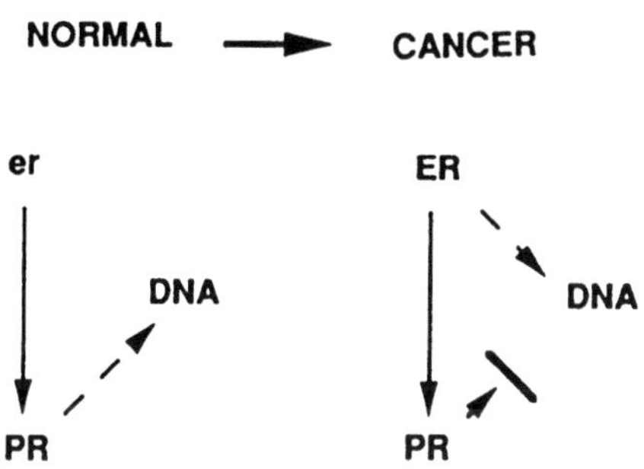


**Fig. 1.** Upregulation of oestrogen receptor (ER) as a potential mechanism for changing steroid sensitivity during human mammary carcinogenesis. In normal cells, low levels of oestrogen receptor (er) can upregulate progesterone receptor (PR) which in the presence of a progestin increases DNA synthesis. Possibly, er may have a small, direct effect on DNA (not shown). Upregulation of ER in cancer cells increases/changes their sensitivity to oestrogen; additional changes alter progestin responses. This block may not be complete (not shown)

This is known to occur in rat models, although in that situation progestin effects are the opposite [3,19] of those being hypothesised here for human mammary carcinogenesis. A possible mechanism for such a switch is mentioned below.

Effects of progestins on established breast cancer are poorly defined. Pharmacologic levels of progestins can induce regressions in advanced breast cancer [9], whilst physiological levels can inhibit growth of human breast cancer cell lines [26,27]. However, all of the latter experiments were performed in the oestrogenic environment of phenol red; recent data obtained in the absence of phenol red indicate that progestins can have a weak proliferative activity [28,29]. There are two conflicting reports [26,28] on the actions in cell culture of the antiprogestin RU486 in the absence of oestrogen.

### Altered Steroid Sensitivity Due to Progression

The mitogenic effect of oestradiol on breast cancer cells is proven and there must therefore be a change in steroid sensitivity from

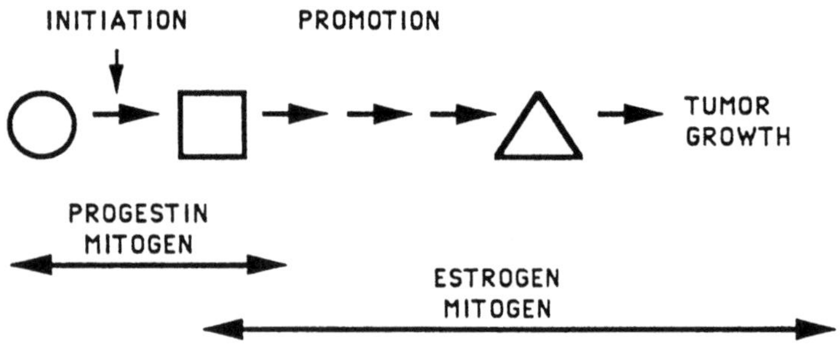


**Fig. 2.** A model of progestin and oestrogen involvement in human mammary carcinogenesis. An hypothetical switch in steroid sensitivity occurs during progression and is depicted here as occurring at an early stage of promotion; it could occur at a later stage. Other features of the model are listed in Table 1

progestin to oestrogen somewhere along the progression pathway. One candidate mechanism for such a change might be the upregulation of oestrogen receptor (ER) that occurs during progression [30,31] (Fig. 1). It is now clear from molecular biological studies that steroid sensitivity is markedly dependent on the number of receptors per cell [32,33]. Thus, the increased ER content of some breast tumours relative to that seen in normal mammary epithelium could result in heightened oestrogen sensitivity. This cannot be the only change, otherwise one would predict that progestins should be strongly mitogenic for the cancer cells, which is not the case. However, recent data with human breast cancer cell lines indicate that progestins can retain weak proliferative activity under certain conditions in such advanced breast cancer cells [28,29]. Thus, the effects of physiological levels of progestagens on breast cancer cell proliferation are unclear, although pharmacologic levels are undoubtedly cytotoxic [9].

## Conclusions

Sufficient doubts exist to question the view that oestrogens alone adversely influence human mammary carcinogenesis particularly in its early stages. The alternative oestrogen plus progestagen view warrants more attention and one possible model is illustrated in Figure 2, with its main features listed in Table 1. Two essential differences from the oestrogen-alone model are that progestins are not benign or even beneficial agents and that the steroid effect varies with stage of neoplastic process. This model is compatible with the existing data outlined above.

None of the points and counterpoints made in this chapter lead to firm conclusions and more data are urgently required to establish the validity or otherwise of many of the arguments presented. The possibility of progestins having adverse effects on early stages of human breast carcinogenesis deserves further consideration as it has important consequences. The influence of the contraceptive pill is a case in point, but discussions on ways of preventing breast cancer are taking place; these are largely based on the oestrogen model [34,35,36]. These should continue, but additional thinking about anti-progestins is called for as they may have inherent advantages over antioestrogens, whilst the use of progestins for this purpose may be counterproductive. At the cell biological and biochemical level, oestrogens have dominated thinking and practical effort; progestins warrant at least equal attention.

**Table 1.** Main features of an oestrogen plus progestin model of human mammary carcinogenesis

| | |
|---|---|
| 1 | Progestins, by their mitogenic effect, increase the probability of successful initiation/early promotion events |
| 2 | Oestrogens, by inducing progesterone receptor, increase the mitogenic potency of progestins |
| 3 | A change in steroid sensitivity accompanies progression so that oestrogens become mitogenic for established cancer cells and possibly for preneoplastic cells |

## REFERENCES


1 Henderson BE, Ross R and Bernstein L: Estrogens as a cause of human cancer. Cancer Res 1988 (48):246-253

2 Vessey MP: The involvement of oestrogen in the development and progression of breast disease: epidemiological evidence. Proc Royal Soc Edin, 1989 (95B):35-48

3 Fowler EH: Progesterone and synthetic progestins: their biological activity and role in neoplasia. In: Kellen JA, Hilf R (eds) Influences of Hormones in Tumor Development. CRC Press, Florida, 1979 pp 45-84

4 Welsch CW: Hormones and murine mammary tumorigenesis: an historical view. In: Leung BS (ed) Hormonal Regulation of Mammary Tumors. Eden Press, Montreal 1982 pp 1-29

5 Darbre PD and King RJB: Steroid hormone regulation of cultured breast cancer cells. In: Lippman ME, Dickson RB (eds) Breast Cancer: Cellular and Molecular Biology. Kluwer Academic, Boston 1988 pp 307-341

6 Dickson RB and Lippman ME: Breast Cancer: Cellular and Molecular Biology. Kluwer Academic, Boston 1988 pp 119-165

7 Mouridsen HT: Endocrine treatment of advanced breast cancer. In: Cavalli F (ed) Endocrine Therapy of Breast Cancer. European School of Oncology Monograph. Springer-Verlag, Berlin 1986 pp 79-90

8 King RJB and Whitehead MI: Assessment of the potency of orally administered progestins in women. Fertil Steril 1986 (46):1062-1066

9 Horwitz KB, Wei LL, Sedlacek SM and D'Arville CN: Progestin action and progesterone receptor structure in human breast cancer: a review. Recent Prog Horm Res 1985 (41):249-316

10 Key JA and Pike MC: The role of oestrogens and progestagens in the epidemiology and prevention of breast cancer. Eur J Cancer Clin Oncol 1988 (24):29-43

11 Going JJ, Anderson TJ, Battersby S and MacIntyre CCA: Proliferative and secretory activity in human breast during natural and artificial menstrual cycles. Am J Pathol 1988 (130):193-203

12 Anderson TJ, Battersby S, King RJB, McPherson K and Going JJ: Oral contraceptive use influences resting breast proliferation. Hum Pathol 1989 (20):1139-1144

13 Meyer JS: Cell proliferation in normal human breast ducts, fibroadenomas and other duct hyperplasias, measured by nuclear labelling with tritiated thymidine: effects of menstrual phase, age, and oral contraceptive hormones. Human Pathol 1977 (8):67-81

14 Longacre TA and Bartow SA: A correlative morphologic study of human breast and endometrium in the menstrual cycle. Am J Surg Pathol 1986 (10):382-293

15 Potten CS, Watson RJ, Williams GT, Tickle S, Roberts SA, Harris M and Howell A: The effect of age and menstrual cycle upon proliferative activity of the normal human breast. Br J Cancer 1988 (58):163-170

16 Chilvers C, McPherson K, Peto J, Pike MC and Vessey MP: Oral contraceptive use and breast cancer risk in young women. Lancet 1989 (i):973-982

17 Schlesselman JJ: Cancer of the breast and reproductive tract in relation to use of oral contraceptives. Contraception 1989 (40):1-38

18 Bergkvist L, Adami H-O, Persson I, Hoover R and Schairer C: The risk of breast cancer after estrogen and estrogen-progestin replacement. N Engl J Med 1989 (321):293-297

19 Russo J, Tay LK and Russo IH: Differentiation of the mammary gland and susceptibility to carcinogenesis. Breast Cancer Res Treat 1981 (2):5-73

20 Korenman SG: Reproductive endocrinology and breast cancer in women. Banbury Reports 1981 (8):71-85

21 Apter D and Vihko R: Early menarche, a risk factor for breast cancer indicates early onset of ovulatory cycles. J Clin Endo Metab 1983 (57):82-86

22 Henderson BE, Ross RK, Judd HL, Krailo MD and Pike MC: Do regular ovulatory cycles increase breast cancer risk? Cancer 1985 (56):1206-1208

23 Mauvais-Jarvis P, Kuttenn F and Gompel A: Antiestrogen action of progesterone in breast cancer. Breast Cancer Res Treat 1986 (8):179-188

24 McManus MJ and Welsch CW: The effect of estrogen, progesterone, thyrosine, and human placental lactogen on DNA synthesis of human breast ductal epithelium maintained in athymic nude mice. Cancer 1984 (54):1920-1927

25 King, RJB and Cowan DM: The effect of dimethylbenzanthracene on the incorporation of [3H] thymidine into DNA of rat mammary gland and uterus. Eur J Cancer 1970 (6):111-113

26 Gill PG, Vignon F, Bardon S, Derocq D and Rochefort H: Difference between R5020 and the antiprogestin RU486 in antiproliferative effects on human breast cancer cells. Breast Cancer Res Treat 1987 (10):37-45

27 Sutherland RI, Hall RE, Pang YN, Musgrove EA and Clarke CL: Effect of medroxyprogesterone acetate

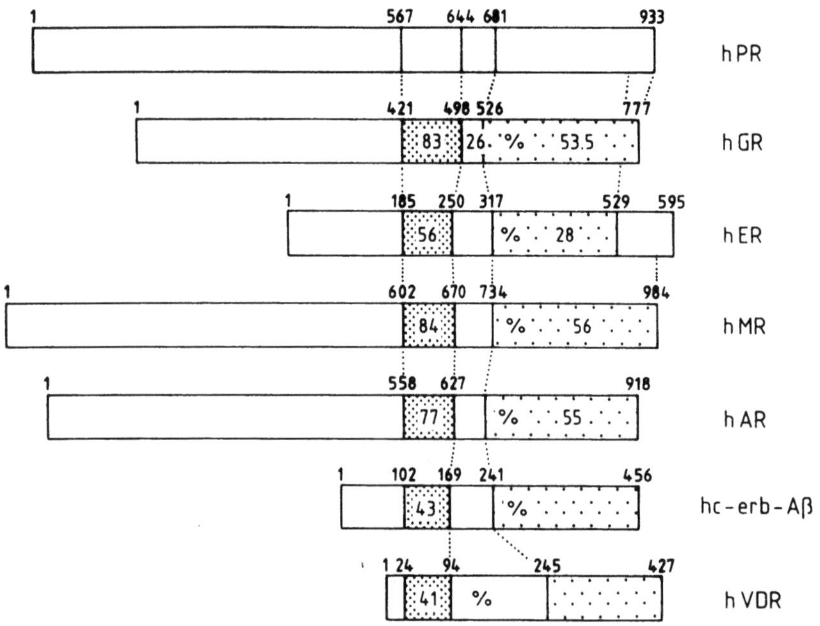


**Fig. 1.** Schematic comparison between human progesterone (hPR), glucocorticoid (hGR), oestrogen (hER), mineralocorticoid (hMR), androgen (hAR), thyroid (hc-erb-aß) and vitamin D (h VDR) receptors.
Receptors are aligned through their DNA binding domain (dark boxes). Steroid binding domains are shown by dotted boxes. Percent homology to progesterone receptor is indicated

does not bind to the chick receptor and is inactive as a progesterone antagonist in this species. The N-terminal half of the receptors is the most variable region, both in length and in amino-acid sequence. It contains some transcription modulating sequences, and it is found to be the major antigenic region when epitopes recognised by monoclonal antibodies against glucocorticoid and progesterone receptors are mapped [18].

## Subfamilies Among Nuclear Receptors. Relationship with Oncogenes and Anti-Oncogenes

This family of proteins involves not only receptors for steroid hormones but also receptors from derivatives of lipophilic vitamins (vitamin D [19,20] and retinoic acid [21-25]) and thyroid hormones [16,17]. Various morphogenetic and developmental regulators [26-28] or transcription factors [29,30] with no known receptor function have also been described. The fact that these proteins may, especially when modified, play a role as oncogenes and anti-oncogenes, is best exemplified by the history of the discovery of the thyroid and retinoic acid receptors. Avian erythroblastosis virus contains 2 oncogenes: v-*erb*-B, which is a truncated derivative of the EGF receptor, and v-*erb*-A, whose function was unknown until the glucocorticoid receptor had been cloned and sequenced. It was then found by random computer search that the DNA binding domain of the receptor had a marked similarity to a region of v-*erb*-A [31]. It was thus suspected that the latter might be a viral derivative of a normal cellular gene having some receptor function. This observation led to isolation by cross-hybridisation of the cDNA encoding c-*erb*-A (the normal cellular equivalent of v-*erb*-A). It was subsequently established that c-*erb*-A bound triiodothyronine and was thus the thyroid hormone receptor [16,17]. Several variants of this receptor were later identified and shown to be variably expressed in different tissues [2,32-34]. v-*erb*-A was found to be a non-ligand binding equivalent of c-*erb*-A and to exert an inhibitory action on its biological activity. v-*erb*-A bound to thyroid hormone-responsive elements without eliciting any biological activity [35-37]. It probably opposed crucial effects of thyroid hormones during the differentiation of erythyroid cells. c-*erb*-A may thus be considered as an anti-oncogene since, when its biological activity is inhibited, some target cells become oriented towards a malignant phenotype.

Another line of research which led to similar conclusions regarding the relationship between intranuclear receptors and cancer was the search in human hepatomas for insertion sites of hepatitis virus DNA. In one patient, such a site was cloned and sequenced and found to encode a polypeptide homologous to the DNA binding domain of steroid receptors [38]. The cloning of the corresponding cDNA led to the isolation of the proto-oncogene (normal cellular equivalent of the oncogene), which was subsequently found to bind retinoic acid. Two other types of retinoic acid receptors were later described [21-25]. It is likely that insertion of hepatitis virus DNA had activated the retinoic acid receptor gene and had led to the synthesis of an abnormal form of the receptor which elicited, at least partially, the malignant transformation of hepatic cells. The modified retinoic acid receptor thus played the role of an oncogene.

The family of nuclear receptors has been further extended by 2 types of observations. Firstly, cross-hybridising cDNA species were cloned and sequenced, showing the characteristic pattern of nuclear receptors, for which, however, the nature of the ligand was unknown [2,39]. These "orphan" receptors await discovery of their function. Secondly, several genetic loci have been located in drosophila which direct various stages of embryological development and for which cloning and sequencing of the corresponding genes has clearly shown that they belong also to the family of intranuclear receptors [26-28]. Since such genes are usually highly conserved during evolution, we may expect, in the near future, their cloning in mammalian cells. The study of their function may be of interest for the understanding of the differentiation and growth of various cell types and thus for the analysis of the mechanisms of their malignant transformation. It is, at present, unknown if the function of these proteins is controlled through the binding of a ligand.

Among this large family of nuclear transcriptional regulators, 2 subgroups may be defined by their very close structural analogy. One involves the receptors for glucocorticoids, progestins, mineralocorticoids and androgens (receptors for steroids having mainly a 3 keto $\Delta$ 4 structure in their A ring). All of these receptors share more than 80% homology in their DNA binding domain. This explains why, in many cases, they can modulate the function of the same hormone-responsive elements. For instance, all stimulate the transcription of Mouse Mammary Virus (MMTV) Long Terminal Repeat (LTR) promoter. The similarity of these receptors is also high in the steroid binding region (>50%), but is totally divergent in the N-terminal domain. Another subgroup involves the different thyroid hormone and retinoic acid receptors. The oestrogen receptor does not belong to any of these subgroups.

## Chromosomal Localisation of Receptor Genes

All nuclear receptors seem to be derived from a common ancestor. It was thus of some surprise to find that they were scattered throughout the genome. For instance, the oestrogen receptor gene was present on chromosome 6q24-27 [40], the progesterone receptor gene on chromosome 11q22-23 [41], the glucocorticoid receptor gene on 5q-q32 [42], etc. Only some of the receptors for retinoic acid and thyroid hormones are clustered in the same regions of chromosomes 3 and 17 [43-45].

Receptor genes are very large, due to the presence of large introns. For instance, the oestrogen receptor gene is over 140 Kb long, and contains 8 exons [46]. An interesting feature is the fact that the two zinc fingers of the DNA binding domain are encoded by separate exons.

The structure of the promoters of the receptors has been described [47], and the mechanisms which direct their hormonal regulation and tissue-specific expression are currently analysed.

## Posttranslational Modifications of the Receptors

Two types of receptor phosphorylation reactions have been described. For oestrogen receptors, Auricchio and coworkers [48] have observed a tyrosine phosphorylation, catalysed by a specific kinase, which seems to be a prerequisite for the receptor to bind the hormone. No similar results have been reported by other groups.

Serine phosphorylations have been observed for progesterone [49,40], glucocorti-

either in frozen [75,76] or in paraffin-embedded sections [77,78] of hormone-dependent cancers, especially breast cancer.

## REFERENCES


1 Godowski PJ and Picard D: How to be both a receptor and a transcription factor. Biochem Pharmacol 1989 (38):3135-3143

2 Evans RM: The steroid and thyroid hormone receptor superfamily. Science 1988 (240):889-895

3 Green S and Chambon P: Nuclear receptors enhance our understanding of transcription regulation. TIG 1988 (4):309-314

4 Hollenberg SM, Weinberger C, Ong ES, Cerelli G, Oro A, Lebo R, Thompson EB, Rosenfeld MG and Evans RM: Primary structure and expression of a functional human glucocorticoid receptor cDNA. Nature 1985 (318):635-641

5 Greene GL, Gilna P, Waterfield M, Baker A, Hort Y and Shine J: Sequence and expression of human estrogen receptor complementary DNA. Science 1986 (231):1150-1154

6 Green S, Walter P, Kumar V, Krust A, Bornert J, Argos P and Chambon P: Human estrogen receptor cDNA: sequence, expression and homology to v-erb-A. Nature 1986 (320):134-139

7 Loosfelt H, Atger M, Misrahi M, Guiochon-Mantel A, Meriel C, Logeat F, Benarous R and Milgrom E: Cloning and sequence analysis of rabbit progesterone-receptor complementary DNA. Proc Natl Acad Sci USA 1986 (83):9045-9049

8 Misrahi M, Atger M, d'Auriol L, Loosfelt H, Meriel C, Fridlansky F, Guiochon-Mantel A, Galibert F and Milgrom E: Complete amino acid sequence of the human progesterone receptor deduced from cloned cDNA. Biochem Biophys Res Commun 1987 (143):740-748

9 Conneely OM, Dobson ADW, Tsai M, Beattie WG, Toft DO, Huckaby CS, Zarucki T, Schrader WT and O'Malley BW: Sequence and expression of a functional chicken progesterone receptor. Mol Endocrinol 1987 (1):515-525

10 Gronemeyer H, Turcotte B, Quirin-Stricker C, Bocquel MT, Meyer ME, Krozowski Z, Jeltsch MM, Lerongo T, Garnier JM, Chambon P: The chicken progesterone receptor: sequence, expression and functional analysis. EMBO J 1987 (6):3985-3994

11 Arriza JL, Weinberger C, Cerelli G, Glaser TM, Handelin BL, Housman DE and Evans RM: Cloning of human mineralocorticoid receptor complementary DNA: Structural and functional kinship with the glucocorticoid receptor. Science 1987 (237):268-275

12 Chang C, Kokontis J and Liao S: Molecular cloning of human and rat complementary DNA encoding androgen receptors. Science 1988 (240):324-326

13 Lubahn DB, Joseph DR, Sar M, Tan J, Higgs HN, Larson RE, French FS and Wilson EM: The human androgen receptor: complementary deoxyribonucleic acid cloning, sequence analysis and gene expression in prostate. Mol Endocrinol 1988 (2):1265-1275

14 Trapman J, Klaassen P, Kuper GGJM, van der Korput JAGM, Faber PW, van Rooij HCJ, Geurts van Kessel A, Voorhorst MM, Mulder E and Brinkmann AO: Cloning, structure and expression of a cDNA encoding for human androgen receptor. Biochem Biophys Res Commun 1988 (153):241-248

15 Tilley WD, Marcelli M, Wilson JD and McPhaul MJ: Characterization and expression of a cDNA encoding the human androgen receptor. Proc Natl Acad Sci USA 1989 (86):327-331

16 Sap J, Munoz A, Damm K, Goldberg Y, Ghysdael J, Lentz A, Beug H and Vennstrom B: The c-erb-A protein is a high affinity receptor for thyroid hormone. Nature 1986 (324):635-640

17 Weinberger C, Thompson CC, Org ES, Lebo R, Gruol DJ and Evans RM: The c-erb-A gene encodes a thyroid hormone receptor. Nature 1986 (324):641-646

18 Lorenzo F, Jolivet A, Loosfelt H, Vu Hai MT, Brailly S, Perrot-Applanat M and Milgrom E: A rapid method of epitope mapping. Application to the study of immunogenic domains and to the characterization of various forms of rabbit progesterone receptor. Eur J Biochem 1988 (176):53-60

19 McDonnell DP, Mangelsdorf DJ, Pike JW, Haussler MR and O'Malley BW: Molecular cloning of complementary DNA encoding for the avian receptor for vitamin D. Science 1987 (235):1214-1217

20 Baker AR, McDonnell DP, Hughes M, Crisp TM, Mangelsdorf DJ, Haussler MR, Pike JW, Shine J and O'Malley BW: Cloning and expression of full-length cDNA encoding human vitamin D receptor. Proc Natl Acad Sci USA 1988 (85):3294-3298

21 Brand N, Petkovich M, Krust A, Chambon P, de The H, Marchi A, Tiollais P and Dejean A: Identification of a second human retinoic acid receptor. Nature 1988 (332):850-853

22 Petkovich M, Brand NJ, Kurst A and Chambon P: A human retinoic acid receptor which belongs to the family of nuclear receptors. Nature 1987 (330):444-450

23 Giguere V, Ong ES, Segui P and Evans EM: Identification of a receptor for the morphogen retinoic acid. Nature 1987 (330):624-629

24 Krust A, Kastner Ph, Petkovich M, Zelent A and Chambon P: A third human retinoic acid receptor, hRAR-gamma. Proc Natl Acad Sci USA 1989 (86):5310-5314

25 Dolle P, Ruberte E, Kastner P, Petkovich M, Stoner CM, Gudas LJ and Chambon P: Differential expression of genes encoding alpha, beta and gamma retinoic acid receptors and CRABP in the developing limbs of the mouse. Nature 1989 (342):702-705

26 Nauber U, Pankratz MJ, Kienlin A, Seifert E, Klemm U and Jäckle H: Abdominal segmentation of the Drosophila embryo requires a hormone receptor-like protein encoded by the gap gene knirps. Nature 1988 (336):489-492

27 Oro AE, Ong ES, Margolis JS, Posakony JW, McKeown M and Evans RM: The Drosophila gene knirps-related is a member of the steroid-receptor gene superfamily. Nature 1988 (336):493-496

28 Rothe M, Nauber U and Jäckle H: Three hormone receptor-like Drosophila genes encode an identical DNA-binding finger. EMBO J 1989 (8):3087-3094
29 Wang LH, Tsai SY, Cook RG, Beattie WG, Tsai MJ and O'Malley B: COUP transcription factor is a member of the steroid receptor superfamily. Nature 1989 (340):163-166
30 Ryseck RP, MacDonald-Bravo H, Mattei MG, Ruppert S and Bravo R: Structure, mapping and expression of a growth factor inducible gene encoding a putative nuclear hormonal binding receptor. EMBO J 1989 (8):3327-3335
31 Weinberger C, Hollenberg SM, Rosenfeld MG and Evans RM: Domain structure of human glucocorticoid receptor and its relationship to the v-erb-A oncogene product. Nature 1985 (318):670-672
32 Thompson CC, Weinberger C, Lebo R and Evans RM: Identification of a novel thyroid hormone receptor expressed in the mammalian central nervous system. Science 1987 (237):1610-1614
33 Benbrook D and Pfahl M: A novel thyroid hormone receptor encoded by a cDNA clone from a human testis library. Science 1987 (238):788-791
34 Bradley DJ, Young III WS and Weinberger C: Differential expression of alpha and beta thyroid hormone receptor genes in rat brain and pituitary. Proc Natl Acad Sci USA 1989 (86):7250-7254
35 Damm K, Thompson CC and Evans RM: Protein encoded by v-erb-A functions as a thyroid-hormone receptor antagonist. Nature 1989 (339):593-597
36 Sap J, Munoz A, Schmitt J, Stunnenberg H and Vennström B: Repression of transcription mediated at a thyroid hormone response element by the v-erb-A oncogene product. Nature 1989 (340):242-244
37 Gandrillon O, Jurdic P, Pain B, Desbois C, Madjar JJ, Moscovici MG, Moscovici C and Samarut J: Expression of the v-erb-A product, an altered nuclear hormone receptor, is sufficient to transform erythrocytic cells in vitro. Cell 1989 (58):115-121
38 Dejean A, Bougueleret L, Grzeschik KH and Tiollais P: Hepatitis B virus DNA interaction in a sequence homologous to v-erb-A and steroid receptor genes in a hepatocellular carcinoma. Nature 1986 (322):70-72
39 Chang C, Kokontis J, Acakpo-Satchivi L, Liao S, Takeda H and Chang Y: Molecular cloning of new human TR2 receptors: a class of steroid receptor with multiple ligand-binding domains. Biochem Biophys Res Commun 1989 (165):735-741
40 Gosden JR, Middleton PG and Rout D: Localisation of the human oestrogen receptor gene to chromosome 6q24-27 by in situ hybridization. Cytogenet Cell Genet 1986 (43):218-220
41 Rousseau-Merck MF, Misrahi M, Loosfelt H, Milgrom E and Berger R: Localization of the human progesterone receptor gene to chromosome 11q22-11q23. Human Genet 1987 (77):280-282
42 Francke U and Foellmer BE: The glucocorticoid receptor gene is in 5q-q32. Genomics 1989 (4):610-612
43 Mattei MG, Petkovich M, Mattei JF, Brand N and Chambon P: Mapping of the human retinoic acid receptor to the q21 band of chromosome 17. Human Genet 1988 (80):186-188
44 Mattei MA, de The H, Mattei JF, Marchio A, Tiollais P and Dejean A: Assignment of the human hap retinoic acid receptor RAR beta gene to the p24 band of chromosome 3. Human Genet 1988 (80):189-190
45 Rider SH, Gorman PA, Shipley JM, Moore G, Vennstrom B, Solomon E and Sheer D: Localization of the oncogene c-erb-A2 to human chromosome 3. Ann Human Genet 1987 (51):153-160
46 Ponglikitnongkol M, Green S and Chambon P: Genomic organization of the human estrogen receptor gene. EMBO J 1988 (7):3385-3388
47 Misrahi M, Loosfelt H, Atger M, Meriel C, Zerah V, Dessen P and Milgrom E: Organization of the entire rabbit progesterone receptor mRNA and of the promoter and 5' flanking region of the gene. Nucleic Acids Res 1988 (16):5459-5472
48 Auricchio F: Phosphorylation of steroid receptors. J Steroid Biochem 1989 (32):613-622
49 Logeat F, Le Cunff M, Pamphile R and Milgrom E: The nuclear-bound form of the progesterone receptor is generated through a hormone-dependent phosphorylation. Biochem Biophys Res Commun 1985 (131):421-427
50 Sullivan WP, Madden BJ, McCornick DJ and Toft D: Hormone-dependent phosphorylation of the avian progesterone receptor. J Biol Chem 1988 (263):14717-14273
51 Orti E, Mendel DB, Smith LI and Munck A: Agonist-dependent phosphorylation and nuclear dephosphorylation of glucocorticoid receptors in intact cells. J Biol Chem 1989 (264):9728-9731
52 Logeat F, Le Cunff M, Rauch M, Brailly S and Milgrom E: Characterization of a casein kinase which interacts with the rabbit progesterone receptor. Differences with the in vivo hormone-dependent phosphorylation. Eur J Biochem 1987 (170):51-57
53 Bailly A, Le Page C, Rauch M and Milgrom E: Sequence-specific DNA binding of the progesterone receptor to the uteroglobin gene: effects of hormone, antihormone and receptor phosporylation. EMBO J 1986 (5):3235-3241
54 Evans RM and Hollenberg SM: Zinc fingers: Gilt by association. Cell 1988 (52):1-3
55 Freedman LP, Luisi BF, Korszun RZ, Basavappa R, Sigler PB and Yamamoto KR: The function and structure of the metal coordination sites within the glucocorticoid receptor DNA binding domain. Nature 1988 (334):543-546
56 Beato M: Gene regulation by steroid hormones. Cell 1989 (56):335-344
57 Kumar V and Chambon P: The estrogen receptor binds tightly to its responsive element as a ligand-induced homodimer. Cell 1988 (55):145-156
58 Tsai SY, Carlstedt-Duke J, Weigel NL, Dahlamn K, Gustafsson JA, Tsai MJ and O'Malley BW: Molecular interactions of steroid hormone receptor with its enhancer element: Evidence for receptor dimer formation. Cell 1988 (55):361-369
59 Guiochon-Mantel A, Loosfelt H, Lescop P, Sar S, Atger M, Perrot-Applanat M and Milgrom E: Mechanisms of nuclear localization of the progesterone receptor: Evidence for interaction between monomers. Cell 1989 (57):1147-1154

60 Theveny B, Bailly A, Rauch C, Delain E and Milgrom E: Association of DNA-bound progesterone receptors. Nature 1987 (329):79-81
61 Schule R, Muller M, Kaltschmidt C and Renkawitz R: Many transcription factors interact synergistically with steroid receptors. Science 1988 (242):1418-1420
62 Drouin J, Charron J, Gagner JP, Jeannotte L, Nemer M, Plante RK and Wrange O: The pro-opiomelanocortin gene: a model for negative regulation of transcription by glucocorticoids. J Cell Biochem 1987 (35):293-304
63 Akerblom IE, Slater EP, Beato M, Baxter JD and Mellon PL: Negative regulation by glucocorticoids through interference with a cAMP responsive enhancer. Science 1988 (241):350-353
64 Becker PB, Gloss B, Schmid W, Strähle U and Schutz G: In vivo protein-DNA interactions in a glucocorticoid response element require the presence of the hormone. Nature 1986 (324):686-688
65 Willmann T and Beato M: Steroid-free glucocorticoid receptor binds specifically to mouse mammary tumor virus DNA. Nature 1986 (324):688-691
66 Klein-Hitpass L, Tsai SY, Weigel NL, Allan GF, Riley D, Rodriguez R, Schrader WT, Tsai MJ and O'Malley BW: The progesterone receptor stimulates cell-free transcription by enhancing the formation of a stable preinitiation complex. Cell 1990 (60):247-257
67 Catelli MG, Binart N, Jung-Testas I, Renoir JM, Baulieu EE, Feramisco JR and Welch WJ: The common 90-kD protein component of non-transformed "8S" steroid receptors is a heat-shock protein. EMBO J 1985 (4):3131-3135
68 Mendel DB, Bodwell JE, Gametchu B, Harrison RW and Munck A: Molybdate-stabilized nonactivated glucocorticoid-receptor complexes contain a 90-kDa non-steroid binding phosphoprotein that is lost on activation. J Biol Chem 1986 (261):3758-3763
69 Schuh S, Yonemoto W, Brugge J, Bauer VJ, Riehl RM, Sullivan WP and Toft DO: A 90,000-dalton binding protein common to both steroid receptors and the Rous sarcoma virus transforming protein pp60$^{v\text{-}src}$. J Biol Chem 1985 (260):14292-14296
70 Guiochon-Mantel A, Loosfelt H, Ragot T, Atger M, Perricaudet M and Milgrom E: Receptors bound to antiprogestin form abortive complexes with hormone responsive elements. Nature 1988 (336):695-698
71 King WJ and Geene GL: Monoclonal antibodies localize oestrogen receptor in the nuclei of target cells. Nature 1984 (307):745-747
72 Perrot-Applanat M, Logeat F, Groyer-Picard MT and Milgrom E: Immunocytochemical study of mammalian progesterone receptor using monoclonal antibodies. Endocrinology 1985 (116):1473-1484
73 Perrot-Applanat M, Groyer-Picard MT, Logeat F and Milgrom E: Ultrastructural localization of the progesterone receptor by an immunogold method: Effect of hormone administration. J Cell Biol 1986 (102):1191-1199
74 Picard D and Yamamoto KR: Two signals mediate hormone-dependent nuclear localization of the glucocorticoid receptor. EMBO J 1987 (6):3333-3340
75 King WL, DeSombre ER, Jensen EV and Greene GL: Comparison of immunocytochemical and steroid binding assays for estrogen receptor in human breast tumors. Cancer Res 1985 (45):293-304
76 Perrot-Applanat M, Groyer-Picard MT, Lorenzo F, Jolivet A, Vu Hai MT, Pallud C, Spyratos F and Milgrom E: Immunocytochemical study with monoclonal antibodies to progesterone receptor in human breast tumors. Cancer Res 1987 (47):2652-2661
77 Shintaku IP and Said JW: Detection of estrogen receptors with monoclonal antibodies in routinely processed formalin-fixed paraffin sections of breast carcinoma. Am J Clin Pathol 1987 (87):161-167
78 Perrot-Applanat M, Groyer-Picard MT, Vu Hai MT, Pallud C, Spyratos F and Milgrom E: Immunocytochemical staining of progesterone receptor in paraffin sections of human breast cancers. Am J Pathol 1989 (135):457-468

# Prognostic Factors in Breast Cancer

Jan G.M. Klijn and John A. Foekens

Division of Endocrine Oncology, Dr. Daniël den Hoed Cancer Centre, Groene Hilledijk 301, 3075 AE Rotterdam, The Netherlands

New directions in research regarding adjuvant treatment of patients with early breast cancer concerns (potential) new treatment modalities and better selection of high- and low-risk patients. In the current discussion on the application of systemic adjuvant therapy in primary breast cancer, identification of high- and low-risk patients is a major issue [1]. Several classical (Table 1) and second-generation prognostic factors (proliferation rate, DNA ploidy, oncogenes, growth factor receptors, and some glycoproteins) are used for making therapeutic decisions [2]. At present, more than 60 prognostic parameters have been reported and can be classified into 4 main groups: patient characteristics, blood parameters, tumour characteristics and response to therapy (Table 2).

## Patient Characteristics

### *Race*

In a retrospective analysis of a population-based prospective follow-up study including 2,322 white and 536 black women, black women appeared to have a worse prognosis [3]. Overall, the cumulative percentage of survivors at 3 years was 83% among whites compared with 71% among blacks. The racial difference in survival was greatest among women with advanced disease, and a higher proportion of black women with advanced disease did not receive surgery. Even when the type of surgery and stage of disease were controlled, race was a significant prognostic factor. On the other hand, in a smaller study including 646 patients, race did not appear an independent prognostic factor [4].

### *Age*

The possible prognostic influence of age at diagnosis has remained a matter of continuing controversy. Age appeared to be a significant predictor of survival, depending on mode of evaluation. Most studies using linear regression analysis or multivariate analysis of several modern prognostic factors did not find such a predictive value [4], as in our experience [5]. However, in our previous detailed study on the influence of age [6], the presence of a strong non-monotonous variation in hazard rates was striking, showing the best prognosis in the age groups 40-50 and 60-70

**Table 1.** Classical prognostic factors in primary breast cancer

| | | |
|---|---|---|
| 1) | TNM status | - tumour size<br>- lymph node status<br>- distant metastases |
| 2) | Age, menopausal status | |
| 3) | Histopathology | - mitotic grade<br>- nuclear grade<br>- histological grade |
| 4) | Steroid receptor status (ER,PR) | |

**Table 2.** Classification of prognostic factors in breast cancer

**A. Patient characteristics:**
- race
- age
- menopausal status
- performance status
- metabolic disease

**B. Variables determined in blood:**
- tumour marker levels (CEA, CA15-3)
- haemoglobin, alkaline phosphatase, liver function tests
- Fc$\gamma$R on mononuclear cells
- hormone levels

**C. Tumour characteristics:**
1. histological features: type, grade, vascular invasion, necrosis
2. stage (TNM), bone marrow micrometastases
3. cytoplasmatic and nuclear steroid receptors: ER, PR, AR, vit D-R
4. membrane receptors for hormones and growth factors:
    - LHRH-R
    - PRL-R
    - IGF-1-R
    - EGF-R
    - TGF-beta-R
    - SS-R
5. enzymes, proteins and other cytoplasmatic factors:
    - human milk fat globule antigens (HMFG-1)
    - prostaglandin levels
    - plasminogen activator expression
    - tyrosine kinase activities
    - aromatase activity
    - haptoglobin-related protein (Hpr) epitope expression
    - cathepsin D
    - heat shock proteins
    - pS2 protein
    - growth factor content (EGF, TGF-alpha and beta, IGF-1)
6. chromosomal abnormalities:
    - cytogenetic
    - ploidy
    - amplification, (over)expression of oncogenes (HER-2/neu, C-ErbB-2, int-2, ras, C-myc)
    - deletion of suppressor genes (Rb gene)
7. cell proliferation indices:
    - labelling index
    - S-phase fraction
    - Ki-67 antigen
8. clonogenicity
9. immunological phenotypes

**D. Response to treatment**

years for relapse rate, survival from relapse and overall survival. Young patients (<40 years) had the worst prognosis, as confirmed by Fourquet et al [7]. Comparable results were found in a Swedish study, with an exception for the age group 60 through 69 [8]. In a series of 2,170 consecutive patients from Milan and Houston, age appeared also an independent prognostic factor [9].

### *Menopause*

There is also no agreement on the prognostic value of menopause. In our multivariate analysis, menopausal status only appears to be an independent prognostic factor with respect to relapse rate, but not for overall survival or survival from relapse [6]. With respect to adjuvant therapy, premenopausal women benefit especially from chemotherapy and postmenopausal women from endocrine therapy [10].

### *Performance Status and Other Diseases*

A general phenomenon in cancer patients is that patients in poor physical condition (Karnofsky index, WHO scale) have a worse prognosis compared to patients in good condition. Metabolic diseases may also influence the prognosis of breast cancer patients [11].

## Parameters Measured in Blood

Blood parameters such as low haemoglobin levels, leucoerythroblastic blood cell picture, high alkaline phosphatase activity, high LDH activity and disturbed liver function test indicate a poor prognosis related with high tumour burden in bone (marrow) and liver. Carcinoembryonic antigen (CEA) or CA 15-3 elevation becomes more frequent with increasing stage, increasing tumour bulk, and with bone and visceral metastases [12,13]. Perioperative CEA determination has limited ability to define a small group of patients with increased risk of relapse, but CEA and CA 15-3 levels frequently increase around the time of clinical disease progresssion [12,13].
Patients with carcinomas have elevated levels of Fc receptors for IgG (FcτR) on their peripheral blood mononuclear cells [14]. In patients with metastatic breast cancer, high FcτR levels indicated a worse prognosis.
Increased plasma concentrations of growth stimulatory hormones may indicate poor prognosis. In patients with early or metastatic breast cancer, hyperprolactinaemia is an unfavourable prognostic factor with respect to treatment response and survival [15-17]. In addition, hyperprolactinaemia appeared frequently to precede tumour relapse and to be present in patients at time of tumour progression. Increased growth hormone levels also have been demonstrated in breast cancer patients [18] and may indicate a worse prognosis in patients with hormone-dependent tumours [19]. Some prognostic value can be ascribed to tumoural lactotrophic receptors [20,21].

## Tumour Characteristics

### *Histological Features*

Tumour type, tumour shape, grade (mitotic, nuclear, histological), tumour necrosis, vascular infiltration, and presence of inflammatory response are important prognostic variables [2,4,5,22-26]. Fisher et al. found in their study that nuclear grade was the most important single marker of outcome [22]. Mitotic grade also had an independent prognostic discriminative effect within subgroups determined by tumour size, lymph node and receptor status, but predictions of time to recurrence or death were considerably more accurate when used together with the other prognostic parameters [4,25]. Marked confluent tumour necrosis was associated with a greater risk of mortality than minimal or no necrosis [26].

### *Stage*

Tumour size, lymph node status and the presence of metastatic disease are important

analogues can inhibit the growth of human breast cancer cells *in vitro* [56] and in animals [57]. In the first study on the relationship with survival [5], we demonstrated that patients with SS-R-positive tumours have a significantly better 5-year disease-free survival than patients with SS-R-negative tumours, namely, 82% versus 46% (p=0.04).

## Enzymes, Proteins and Other Cytoplasmatic Factors

Several factors determined in the cytoplasma and organelles of tumour cells have been found to have prognostic value in breast cancer.

The median survival of patients with tumours that stained for human milk fat globule antigens (HMFG-1) in more than 30% of cells was 36 months; with no cells stained, the median survival was 11 months (p <0.0001) [58].

There is no agreement on the relationship of tumour prostaglandin levels to early recurrence [59].

Plasminogen activator (PA) expression seemed to be related to ER and EGF-R status [45,60] in human primary breast cancers. PA is an oestrogen-inducible enzyme. Considerable evidence suggests that the PA/plasmin system plays a role in the development and metastatic spread of tumours, a role that is likely to involve the degradation of matrix and basement membrane proteins by plasmin or plasmin-activated proteases. Harris found that the lack of tPA appears to be associated with an aggressive group of tumours and that EGF-R might have a role in suppressing tPA secretion [45].

Cancers of the breast show considerably higher tyrosine kinase activity in both membrane and cytosol fractions, compared to benign tumours, which showed increased cytosolic activity in comparison to normal breast tissues [61]. There appeared to be a strong association between enhanced expression of tyrosine kinase activity in primary carcinoma cytosols and early systemic relapse.

Also intratumoural aromatase activity (AA) appeared to be a prognostic factor in human breast cancer [62]. Significant AA was found in 91 of 145 (63%) tumour samples. There was no relationship between AA and tumour size, site, nodal status, menopausal status or ER. Tumours with a high grade (poorly differentiated carcinomas) showed significantly higher AA. Time to relapse was marginally shorter in the AA-negative group, but the survival of patients after relapse was significantly longer. No significant difference was found in overall survival between the AA-positive and the AA-negative group.

Recently, haptoglobin-related protein (Hpr) epitope expression measured by immunohistochemical analysis was reported to be an independent prognostic factor [63] in breast cancer. The expression of Hpr epitopes was associated with earlier recurrence. The clinical value was especially important when Hpr-epitope expression was used in combination with PR status.

Of great interest is the Mr 52,000 Cathepsin D, the precursor of a lysosomal protease secreted in excess by breast cancer cells compared with normal mammary cells. This oestrogen-regulated protein displays mitogenic and proteolytic activity, suggesting a role in tumour dissemination. In a first retrospective study inlcuding 396 patients, Thorpe et al. [64] demonstrated that patients with high Cathepsin D concentrations have significantly shorter recurrence-free survival, but only a trend towards shorter overall survival (Table 3). The level of Cathepsin D was not significantly associated with the recognised prognostic factors of age, lymph-node involvement, tumour size or grade. A significant association was found between Cathepsin D concentrations and ER status only in pre/perimenopausal patients, showing a significantly greater proportion of ER-positive patients with high Cathepsin D levels. In node-negative patients, the difference in 5-year disease-free survival between the high- and low-risk group was about 8% in pre/perimenopausal patients and 16% in postmenopausal patients (derived from the figures). In another recent study [65] on 122 patients, the discriminative prognostic value of Cathepsin D appeared more striking, especially in node-negative patients when a cutoff level of 70 pmol/mg protein and metastasis-free survival instead of disease-free survival were used as parameters. Cathepsin D concentrations exceeding 70 pmol/mg protein correlated also with shorter

**Table 3.** Prognostic value of various prognostic factors in patients with node-negative breast cancer

| Ref. | Prognostic factor | No.pts. | % difference between high and low risk in 5-year DFS | 5-year OS |
|---|---|---|---|---|
| 22 | nuclear grade good vs poor | 1157 | 16% | 14% |
| 22 | ER+ vs ER- | 1157 | 8% | 10% |
| 2 | ER+ vs ER- | 1928 | 9% | 9% |
| 2 | tumour size <2 cm vs >5 cm | | 13% | |
| 2,78 | HER-2/Neu | 378 | n.s. | n.s. |
| 72 | diploid vs aneuploid | 395 | 14% | |
| | dipl/low S vs dipl/high S | 253 | 20% | 10% |
| 86 | labelling index | 354 | 18% | 11% |
| 44 | EGF-R+ vs EGF-R- | 24 | ?* | ? |
| 5 | EGF-R+ vs EGF-R- | 77 | n.s. | n.s. |
| 64 | Cathepsin-D, high vs low | 200 | 8-16%° | n.s. (8-20%) ++ |
| 65 | Cathepsin-D high vs low | 68 | ?+ | ? |
| 2 + 2a | idem | 199 | 23% ++ | 22% ++ |
| 66 | Total Cathepsin-D | 159 | n.s. | n.s. |
| 68 | Cathepsin-D (immunohistochem.) | 62 | n.s. | n.s. |
| 69 | $pS_2$+ vs $pS_2$- | 76 | 31% | 13% |

* about 58% at 2 years of follow-up
° pre/perimenopausal - postmenopausal
\+ 70% difference regarding distant metastasis-free survival, "but less strong for DFS"
++ derived from figures
DFS = disease-free survival; OS = overall survival
n.s. = not significant

overall survival (p=0.04). Tandon and McGuire [2], who used another antibody, found a highly significant difference between patients with high and low Cathepsin D levels in 199 node-negative patients, but not in 198 patients with node-positive disease [2a]. In contrast, Namer et al. [66], using an optimal cutoff level of 35 pmol total Cathepsin D plus precursors (TCD) per mg protein in 278 cytosols, found that TCD was a powerful, independent prognostic factor for disease-free and overall survival in node-positive patients, but not in node-negative patients. However, Jäger et al. [67] found no prognostic value in 71 patients, but the follow-up was short. In an immunohistochemical study including 94 patients, Henry et al. [68] demonstrated that positive Cathepsin D immunostaining using a polyclonal antibody was even associated with a significant prognostic advantage in patients with confirmed lymph-node metastasis but not in node-negative patients. Positive staining was associated with ER-positive tumours and with prolonged survival, suggesting that Cathepsin D expression reflects the functional integrity of the oestrogen response pathway. In conclusion, therefore, there is, at present, no agreement regarding optimal techniques, optimal cutoff levels and prognostic value of Cathepsin D on the analogy of EGF-R status.

Other oestrogen-regulated proteins are heat shock proteins. In San Antonio, the level of one such protein (srp27) in cytosols of axillary node-negative breast cancer patients revealed a significant correlation with relapse-free survival [2].

A new prognostic marker is pS2, which is a 84 amino-acid long protein with unknown function and mainly expressed in ER-positive tumours. We found no significant associations between the level of pS2 protein and tumour size, lymph-node status and differentiation grade [69]. Using an optimal cutoff level of 11ng pS2 protein/mg cytosol, we found a very strong prognostic value in both node-negative and node-positive patients, and in ER-positive patients. Five-year overall survival was 97% in $ER^+/PR^+/pS2^+$ patients and only 54% in $ER^+/PR^+/pS2^-$ patients. In node-positive patients, pS2 status discriminates strongly between a good and bad prognosis group with a 54% difference (88 vs. 34%) in overall survival between $pS2^+$ and $pS2^-$ subgroups. In node-negative patients, pS2 appeared to be the most powerful prognosticator, with 31% difference in 5-year disease-free survival between low- and high-risk patients (89% vs. 58%).

Less is known about the prognostic value of tumour cytosolic content of growth factors in contrast to membrane growth factor receptors. We found a negative relationship between IGF-1-like and EGF-like activities on the one hand and steroid receptors (ER,PR) on the other [41]. With respect to transcripts for TGF-α, Coombes et al. [48] found no difference in survival between TGF-α-positive and TGF-α-negative groups. High levels of TGF-ß mRNA were related to a good prognosis.

### *Chromosomal Abnormalities*

Chromosomal abnormalities in breast cancer have been demonstrated on chromosomes 1p, 1q, 3p, 8q, 11p, 11q, 13q, 17p, 17q and 18q. Loss of complete chromosomes is not a frequent event in breast cancer, but allele losses have been described in more than 60% of breast cancers and might be associated with genetically high-risk forms of breast cancer [70,71].

Aneuploidy occurs in more than half of all breast cancers and is related to poor prognosis, especially in node-positive breast cancer [2,72].

Amplification and overexpression of oncogenes or deletion of suppressor genes (Table 2) have been detected in a minority of patients (10-30%) and are frequently related to more aggressive tumours and poor prognosis, but, in general, the prognostic value is weak and mainly present in node-positive patients [51,73-84].

### *Tumour Cell Kinetics*

The proliferative activity of tumours can be measured by the thymidine labelling index [85-88], by DNA flow cytometry (S-phase fraction) [72] or Ki67-index [89,90]. High proliferative activity of tumours clearly seemed to be related to poor prognosis. Clark et al. [72], using 2 prognostic factors together, reported that patients with diploid tumours and low S-phase fraction had a relapse-free survival at 5 years of 90%, compared with 70% for those with diploid tumours and high S-phase fraction. The S-phase fraction was not an important additional predictor of relapse-free survival for patients with aneuploid tumours.

### *Clonogenicity*

Clonogenicity and hormone-induced proliferative response of breast tumours appeared to be good markers of hormonal dependence [91]. Tumours which formed less than 150 colonies per 500,000 cells seeded and which increased their proliferative activity 1.8-fold or more in response to hormones, were the tumours that were likely to respond to endocrine treatments, whereas all other tu-

mours were likely to be refractory to endocrine treatment.
The presence or absence of growth of transplanted pieces of human primary tumours into nude mice also appeared to have prognostic value.

### *Immunological Phenotypes*

(Breast) cancer cells can also be characterised by various immunological phenotypes [92]. However, less is known with respect to their prognostic value.

## Response to Treatment

Response to treatment is an important prognostic parameter. Patients with metastatic disease not responding to hormonal or chemotherapy die within 1/2-1 year, while patients responding to various forms of hormonal therapy and chemotherapy can survive from 3 to more than 10 years.

## Conclusion

As described, there are many prognostic factors in breast cancer. A good discriminative effect between high- and low-risk patients is especially needed in node-negative patients to select patients for systemic adjuvant therapy (Table 3). In our hands, the pS2 protein is one of the most powerful single prognosticators. Combination of prognostic factors can further improve the discriminative efficacy.

## REFERENCES

1 McGuire WL: Adjuvant treatment of node-negative breast cancer. N Engl J Med 1989 (320): 525-527

2 McGuire WL: Prognostic factors for recurrence and survival. In: Educational Booklet American Society of Clinical Oncology, 25th Annual Meeting 1989 pp 89-92

2a Tandon AK, Clark GM, Chamnes GC, Chirgwin JM, McGuire WL: Cathepsin D and prognosis in breast cancer. N Engl J Med 1990 (322):297-302

3 Bain RP, Greenberg RS, Whitaker JP: Racial differences in survival of women with breast cancer. J Chron Dis 1986 (39): 631-642

4 Russo J, Frederick J, Ownby HE, Fine G, Hussain M, Krickstein HI, Robbins TO, Rosenberg B: Predictors of recurrence and survival of patients with breast cancer. J Clin Path 1987 (88): 123-131

5 Foekens JA, Portengen H, van Putten WLJ, Trapman AMAC, Reubi J-C, Alexieva-Figusch J, Klijn JGM: Prognostic value of receptors for insulin-like growth factor 1, somatostatin, and epidermal growth factor in human breast cancer. Cancer Res 1989 (49): 7002-7009

6 Alexieva-Figusch J, van Putten WLJ, Blankenstein MA, Blonk-van der Wijst J, Klijn JGM: The prognostic value and relationships of patient characteristics, estrogen and progestin receptors, and site of relapse in primary breast cancer. Cancer 1988 (61): 758-768

7 Fourquet A, Campana F, Zafrani B, Mosseri V, Vielh P, Durane JC, Vilcoq JR: Prognostic factors of breast recurrence in the conservative management of early breast cancer: a 25-year follow-up. Int J Radiat Oncol Biol Phys 1989 (17): 719-725

8 Adami H-O, Malker B, Meirik O, Persson I, Bergkvist L, Stone B: Age as a prognostic factor in breast cancer. Cancer 1985 (56): 898-902

9 Cascinelli N, Singletary E, Greco M, Ames F, Testori A, Baldini M, Morabito A, Bufalino R, Shallenberger R, Guinee V et al: Long-term survival and prognostic factors for 2170 breast cancer patients treated at two cancer centers (Milan and Houston). Tumori 1989 (75): 123-131

10 Early Breast Cancer Trialists' Collaborative Group: Effects of adjuvant tamoxifen and of cytotoxic therapy on mortality in early breast cancer. N Engl J Med 1988 (319): 1681-1692

11 Beex LVAM: Metabolic diseases influencing prognosis. In: Stoll BA (ed) Breast Cancer: Treatment and Prognosis. Blackwell, Oxford 1986 pp 200-211

12 Beard DB, Haskell CM: Carcinoembryonic antigen in breast cancer, clinical review. Am J Med 1986 (80): 241-245

13 Kerin MJ, McAnena OJ, O'Malley VP, Grimes H, Given HF: CA 15-3: its relationship to clinical stage and progression to metastatic disease in breast cancer. Br J Surg 1989 (76): 838-839

14 Ilfeld D, Barzilay J, Dux Z, Ran M: Correlation of Fcτ receptors on peripheral blood mononuclear cells and survival in patients metastatic cancer. Breast Cancer Res Treatm 1986 (7): 181-186

15 Holtkamp W, Nagel GE, Wander H-E, Rauschecker HF, von Heyden D: Hyperprolactinemia is an indicator of progressive disease and poor prognosis in advanced breast cancer. Int J Cancer 1984 (34): 323-328

16 Dowsett M, McGarrick GE, Harris AL, Coombes RC, Smith IE, Jeffcoate SL: The prognostic significance of hyperprolactinaemia in breast cancer. In: Klijn JGM, Paridaens R, Foekens JA (eds) Hormonal Manipulation of Cancer: Peptides, Growth Factors and New (Anti)Steroidal Agents. Monograph Series of the EORTC, vol 18. Raven Press, New York 1987 pp 175-181

17 Alexieva-Figusch J, de Jong FH, Lamberts SWJ, Planting ASTh, van Gilse HA, Blankenstein MA, Blonk-van der Wijst J, Klijn JGM: Alternating and combined treatment with tamoxifen and progestins in postmenopausal breast cancer. In: Klijn JGM, Paridaens R, Foekens JA (eds) Hormonal Manipulation of Cancer: Peptides, Growth Factors and New (Anti)Steroidal Agents. Monograph Series of the EORTC, vol 18. Raven Press, New York 1987 pp 145-155

18 Emerman JT, Leaky M, Gout PW, Bruchovsky N: Elevated growth hormone levels in sera from breast cancer patients. Horm Metab Res 1985 (17): 421-424

19 Pierrepoint CG, Turkes AO, Walker KJ, Harper ME, Wilson DW, Peeling WB, Griffiths K: Endocrine factors in the treatment of prostatic cancer. In: Schröder FH, Richards B (eds) Therapeutical Principles in Metastatic Prostatic Cancer. Alan R Liss, New York 1985 pp 51-72

20 Waseda N, Kato Y, Imura H, Kurata M: Prognostic value of estrogen and prolactin receptor analysis in human breast cancer. Jpn J Cancer Res 1985 (76): 517-523

21 Bonneterre J, Peyrat JP, Beuscart R, Lefebvre J, Demaille A: Prognostic significance of prolactin receptors (PRL-R) in human breast cancer. Cancer Res 1987 (47): 4724-4728

22 Fisher B, Redmond C, Fisher ER, Caplan R and other contributing National Surgical Adjuvant Breast and

Bowel Project Investigators: Relative worth of estrogen or progesterone receptor and pathologic characteristics of differentiation as indicators of prognosis in node negative breast cancer patients: Findings from NSABBP Project Protocol B-06. J Clin Oncol 1988 (6): 1076-1087

23 Singh L, Wilson AJ, Baum M, Whimster WF, Birch IH, Jackson IM, Lowrey C, Palmer MK: The relationship between histological grade, oestrogen receptor status, events and survival at 8 years in the NATO ("Nolvadex") trial. Br J Cancer 1988 (57): 612-614

24 Davis BW, Gelber RD, Goldhirsch A, Hartmann WH, Locher GW, Reed R, Golouh R, Säve-Söderbergh J, Hollaway L, Russell I, Rudenstam CM, for the Ludwig Breast Cancer Study Group: Prognostic significance of tumor grade in clinical trials of adjuvant therapy for breast cancer with axillary lymph node metastasis. Cancer 1986 (58): 2662-2670

25 Van der Linde JC, Lindeman J, Baak JP, Meijer CJ, Herman CJ: The multivariate prognostic index and nuclear DNA content are independent prognostic factors in primary breast cancer patients. Cytometry 1989 (10): 56-61

26 Shek LLM, Godolphin W: Model for breast cancer survival: relative prognostic roles of axillary nodal status, TNM stage, estrogen receptor concentration, and tumor necrosis. Cancer Res 1988 (48): 5565-5569

27 Clark GM, Sledge GW, Osborne CK, McGuire WL: Survival from first recurrence: relative importance of prognostic factors in 1,015 breast cancer patients. J Clin Oncol 1987 (5): 55-61

28 Coombes RC, Berger U, Mansi J, Redding H, Powles TJ, Neville AM, McKinna A, Nash AG, Gazet J-C, Ford HT, Ormerod M, McDonnell T: Prognostic significance of micrometastases in bone marrow in patients with primary breast cancer. NCI Monogr 1986 (1): 51-53

29 Swennerton KD, Legha SS, Smith T, Hortobagy GN, Gehan EA, Yap HY, Gutterman JU, Blumenschein GR: Prognostic factors in metastatic breast cancer treated with combination chemotherapy. Cancer Res 1979 (39): 1552-1562

30 Foekens JA, Portengen H, van Putten WLJ, Peters HA, Krijnen HLJM, Alexieva-Figusch J, Klijn JGM: Prognostic value of estrogen and progesterone receptors measured by enzym immunoassays in human breast cancer cytosols. Cancer Res 1989 (49): 5823-5828

31 Kinsel LB, Szabo E, Greene GL, Konrath J, Leight GS, McCarty KS: Immunocytochemical analysis of estrogen receptors as a predictor of prognosis in breast cancer patients: comparison with quantitative biochemical methods. Cancer Res 1989 (49):1052-1056

32 Raemaekers JMM, Beex LVAM, Pieters GFFM, Smals AGH, Benraad ThJ, Kloppenborg PWC and the Breast Study Group: Progesterone receptor activity and relapse-free survival in patients with primary breast cancer: the role of adjuvant chemotherapy. Breast Cancer Res Treatm 1987 (9): 191-199

33 Bryan RM, Mercer RJ, Bennett RC, Rennie GC, Lie TH, Morgan FJ: Androgen receptors in breast cancer. Aust N Z J Surg 1984 (54): 2436-2440

34 Colston KW, Berger U, Coombes RC: Possible role for vitamin D in controlling breast cancer cell proliferation. Lancet 1989 (i): 188-191

35 Kaufmann M, Kiesel L, Klinga K, Runnebaum B, Kubli F: Gonadotropin-releasing hormone receptors in human breast carcinoma. In: Abstractbook 4th EORTC Breast Cancer Working Conference 1987: abstr D 2.22

36 Fekete M, Wittliff JL, Schally AW: Characteristics and distribution of receptors for [D-Trp$^6$]-luteinizing-hormone-releasing hormone, somatostatin, epidermal growth factor, and sex steroids in 500 biopsy samples of human breast cancer. J Clin Lab Analysis 1989 (3): 137-141

37 Bonneterre J, Peyrat JP: Prolactin receptors (PRL-R) and breast cancer. Eur J Cancer Clin Oncol 1989 (25): 1121-1122

38 Ben-David M, Wittliff JL, Fekete M, Kadar T, Biran S, Schally AV: Lack of relationship between the levels of prolactin receptors and steroid receptors in women with breast cancer. Biomed Pharmacother 1988 (42):327-334

39 Pekonen F, Partanen S, Mäkinen T, Rutanen E-M: Receptors for epidermal growth factor and insulin-like growth factor 1 and their relation to steroid receptors in human breast cancer. Cancer Res 1988 (48): 1343-1347

40 Peyrat J-P, Bonneterre J, Beuscart R, Djiane J, Demaille A: Insulin-like growth factor 1 receptors in human breast cancer and their relation to estradiol and progesterone receptors. Cancer Res 1988 (48): 6429-6433

41 Foekens JA, Portengen H, Janssen M, Klijn JGM: Insulin-like growth factor 1 receptors and insulin-like growth factor-1-like activity in human primary breast cancer. Cancer 1989 (63): 2139-2147

42 Peyrat J-P, Bonneterre J, Laurent JC, Louchez MM, Amrani S, Leroy-Martin B, Vilain MO, Delobelle A, Demaille A: Presence and characterization of insulin-like growth factor-1 receptors in human

benign breast disease. Eur J Cancer Clin Oncol 1988 (24): 1425-1431

43 Klijn JGM, Foekens JA: Epidermal growth factor receptors (EGF-R) in breast cancer. Ann Oncol 1990 (1): accepted for publication

44 Sainsbury JRC, Farndon JR, Needham GK, Malcolm AJ, Harris AL: Epidermal-growth factor receptor status as predictor of early recurrence of and death from breast cancer. Lancet 1987 (i): 1398-1402

45 Harris AL, Nicholson S: Epidermal growth factor receptors in human breast cancer. In: Lippman ME, Dickson RB (eds) Breast Cancer: Cellular and Molecular Biology. Kluwer Academic Publishers, Boston 1988 pp 93-119

46 Macias A, Azavedo E, Hägerström T, Klintenberg C, Perez R, Skoog L: Prognostic significance of the receptor for epidermal growth factor in human mammary carcinomas. Anticancer Res 1987 (7): 459-464

47 Grimaux M, Romain S, Remvikos Y, Martin PM, Magdelénat H: Prognostic value of epidermal growth factor receptor in node-positive breast cancer. Breast Cancer Res Treatm 1989 (14): 77-90

48 Coombes RC, Murray P, Lugmani Y: The prognostic significance of transcripts for transforming growth factor alpha and beta and epidermal growth factor receptor in primary breast cancer. Eur J Cancer Clin Oncol 1990 (26): February issue, abstr 49 of Second International Symposium on Hormonal Manipulation of Cancer 1990

49 Nicholson S, Sainsbury JRC, Halcrow P, Chambers P, Farndon JR, Harris AL: Expression of epidermal growth factor receptors associated with lack of response to endocrine therapy in recurrent breast cancer. Lancet 1989 (i): 182-185

50 Harris AL: Epidermal growth factor receptor: a marker of early relapse in breast cancer: interactions with Neu. Eur J Cancer Clin Oncol 1989 (26): February issue, abstr 29 of Second International Symposium on Hormonal Manipulation of Cancer 1990

51 Dickson RB, Lippman ME: Control of human breast cancer by estrogen, growth factors, and oncogens. In: Lippman ME, Dickson R (eds) Breast Cancer: Cellular and Molecular Biology. Kluwer Academic Publishers, Boston 1988 pp 119-167

52 Reubi JC, Maurer R, von Werder K, Torhorst J, Klijn JGM, Lamberts SWJ: Somatostatin receptors in human endocrine tumors. Cancer Res 1987 (47): 551-558

53 Papotti M, Macri L, Bussolati G, Reubi JC: Correlative study on neuro-endocrine differentiation and presence of somatostatin receptors in breast carcinomas. Int J Cancer 1989 (43): 365-369

54 Reubi JC, Waser B, Foekens JA, Klijn JGM, Lamberts SWJ, Laissue J: Evaluation of somatostatin receptor incidence and distribution in breast cancer using receptor autoradiography. Int J Cancer 1990 (in press)

55 Reubi JC, Torhorst J: Relationship between somatostatin, EGF- and steroid-hormone receptors in breast cancer. Cancer 1989 (64): 1254-1260

56 Setyono-Han B, Henkelman MS, Foekens JA, Klijn JGM: Direct inhibitory effects of somatostatin (analogues) on the growth of human breast cancer cells. Cancer Res 1987 (47): 1566-1570

57 Szende B, Lapis K, Redding TW, Srkalovic G, Schally AV: Growth inhibition of MXT mammary carcinoma by enhancing programmed cell death (apoptosis) with analogs of LH-RH and somatostatin. Breast Cancer Res Treatm 1989 (14): 307-314

58 Baildam AD, Howell A, Barnes DM, Turnbull L, Sellwood RA: The expression of milk fat globule antigens within human mammary tumours: relationship to steroid hormone receptors and response to endocrine treatment. Eur J Cancer Clin Oncol 1989 (25): 459-467

59 Fulton AM, Ownby HE, Frederick J, Brennan MJ: Relationship of tumor prostaglandin levels to early recurrence in women with primary breast cancer: clinical update. Invasion Metastasis 1986 (6): 83-94

60 Pacheco MM, Brentani MM, Franco EL, Fontelles JA, Chamone DF, Marques LA: Plasminogen activator expression and steroid hormone receptors in female breast cancer: a multifactorial study. Int J Cancer 1988 (41): 798-804

61 Hennipman A, van Oirschot A, Smits J, Rijksen G, Staal GEJ: Tyrosine kinase activity in breast cancer, benign breast disease and normal breast tissue. Cancer Res 1989 (49): 516-521

62 Silva MC, Rowlands MG, Dowsett M, Gusterson B, McKinna JA, Fryatt I, Coombes RC: Intratumoral aromatase as a prognostic factor in human breast carcinoma. Cancer Res 1989 (49): 2588-2591

63 Kuhajda FP, Piantadosi S, Pasternack GR: Haptoglobin-related protein (Hpr) epitopes in breast cancer as a predictor of recurrence of the disease. N Engl J Med 1989 (321): 636-641

64 Thorpe SM, Rochefort H, Garcia M, Freiss G, Christensen IJ, Khalaf S, Paolucci F, Pau B, Rasmussen BB, Rose C: Association between high concentrations of Mr 52,000 cathepsin D and poor prognosis in primary human breast cancer. Cancer Res 1989 (49): 6008-6014

65 Spyratos F, Maudelonde T, Brouillet J-P, Brunet M, Defrenne A, Andrieu C, Hacene K, Desplaces A, Rouëssé J, Rochefort H: Cathepsin D: an

independent prognostic factor for metastasis of breast cancer. Lancet 1989 (ii): 1115-1118
66 Namer M, Ramaioli A, Etienne MC, Fontana JC, Lapalus F, Hery M, Milano G: Prognostic value of total cathepsin D in breast cancer. Eur J Cancer Clin Oncol 1990 (26): February issue, abstr 129 of Second International Symposium on Hormonal Manipulation of Cancer 1990
67 Jäger W, Merkle E, Maloth E, Lang N: Cathepsin D in breast cancer cytosol - follow up after 18 months. Eur J Clin Oncol 1990 (26): February issue, abstr 130 of Second International Symposium on Hormonal Manipulation of Cancer 1990
68 Henry JA, McCarthy AL, Angus B, Westley BR, May FEB, Nicholson S, Cairns J, Harris AL, Horne CHW: Prognostic significance of the estrogen-regulated protein, cathepsin D, in breast cancer. Cancer 1990 (65): 265-271
69 Foekens JA, Rio M-C, Seguin P, van Putten WLJ, Fauque J, Nap M, Klijn JGM, Chambon P: Prediction of relapse and survival in breast cancer patients by pS2 protein status. Cancer Res 1990 (50): in press (June issue)
70 Mackay J, Steel CM, Elder PA, Forrest APM, Evans HJ: Allele loss on short arm of chromosome 17 in breast cancers. Lancet 1988 (ii): 1384-1385
71 Devilee P, Pearson PL, Cornelisse CJ: Allele losses in breast cancer. Lancet 1989 (i): 154
72 Clark GM, Dressler LG, Owens MA, Pounds G, Oldaker T, McGuire WL: Prediction of relapse or survival in patients with node-negative breast cancer by DNA flow cytometry. N Engl J Med 1989 (320): 627-633
73 Ali IU, Lidereau R, Callahan R: Heterogeneity of genetic alterations in primary human breast tumors. In: Lippman ME, Dickson R (Eds) Breast Cancer: Cellular and Molecular Biology. Kluwer Academic Publishers, Boston 1988 pp 25-49
74 Callahan R: Genetic alterations in primary breast cancer. Breast Cancer Res Treat 1989 (13): 191-203
75 Merkel DE, McGuire WL: Oncogenes and cancer prognosis. In: DeVita VT, Hellman S, Rosenberg SA (eds) Important Advances in Oncology. JB Lippincott Company, Philadelphia 1988 pp 103-116
76 Slamon DJ, Clark GM, Wong SG, Levin WJ, Ullrich A, McGuire WL: Human breast cancer: correlation of relapse and survival with amplification of the HER-2/neu oncogene. Science 1987 (235):177-182
77 Slamon DJ, Godolphin W, Jones LA, Holt JA, Wong SG, Keith DE, Levin WJ, Stuart SG, Udove J, Ullrich A, Press MF: Studies of the HER-2/neu proto-oncogene in human breast and ovarian cancer. Science 1989 (244): 707-712
78 Tandon AK, Clark GM, Chamness GC, Ullrich A, McGuire WL: HER-2/neu oncogene protein and prognosis in breast cancer. J Clin Oncol 1989 (7): 1120-1128
79 Van de Vijver MJ, Peterse JL, Mooi WJ, Wisman P, Lomans J, Dalesio O, Nusse R: Neu-protein overexpression in breast cancer: association with comedo-type ductal carcinoma in situ and limited prognostic value in stage II breast cancer. N Engl J Med 1988 (319): 1239-1245
80 Zeillinger R, Kury F, Czerwenka K, Kubista E, Sliutz G, Knogler W, Huber J, Zielinski C, Reiner G, Jakesz R, Staffen A, Reiner A, Wrba F, Spona J: HER-2 amplification, steroid receptors and epidermal growth factor receptor in primary breast cancer. Oncogene 1989 (4): 109-114
81 Wright C, Angus B, Nicholson S, Sainsbury JRC, Cairns J, Gullick WJ, Kelly P, Harris AL, Horne CHW: Expression of C-erbB-2 oncoprotein: a prognostic indicator in human breast cancer. Cancer Res 1989 (49): 2087-2090
82 Adnane J, Gaudray P, Simon M-P, Simony-Lafontaine J, Jeanteur P, Theillet C: Proto-oncogene amplification and human breast tumor phenotype. Oncogene 1989 (4): 1389-1395
83 Tsuda H, Hirobashi S, Shimosato Y et al: Correlation between long-term survival in breast cancer patients and amplification of two putative oncogene-coamplification units: hst-1/int-2 and C-erbB-2/ear-1. Cancer Res 1989 (49): 3104-3108
84 Duffy MJ: Biochemical markers as prognostic indices in breast cancer. Clin Chem 1990 (36): 188-191
85 Meyer JS: Cell kinetics in selection and stratification of patients for adjuvant therapy of breast carcinoma. NCI Monogr 1986 (1): 25-28
86 Silvestrini R, Daidone MG, Valagussa P, Di Fronzo G, Mezzanotte G, Bonadonna G: Cell kinetics as a prognostic indicator in node-negative breast cancer. Eur J Cancer Clin Oncol 1989 (25): 1165-1171
87 Tubiana M, Pejovic MH, Koscielny S, Chavaudra N, Malaise E: Growth rate, kinetics of tumor cell proliferation and long-term outcome in human breast ccancer. Int J Cancer 1989 (44): 17-22
88 Courdi A, Héry M, Dahan E, Gioanni J, Abbes M, Monticelli J, Ettore F, Moll J-L, Namer M: Factors affecting relapse in node-negative breast cancer. A multivariate analysis including the labeling index. Eur J Cancer Clin Oncol 1989 (25): 351-356
89 Charpin C, Andrac L, Vacheret H, Habib MC, Devictor B, Lavaut MN, Toga M: Multiparametric evaluation (SAMBA) of growth fraction (monoclonal

Ki67) in breast carcinoma tissue sections. Cancer Res 1988 (48): 4368-4374

90 Bouzubar N, Walker KJ, Griffiths K, Ellis IO, Elston CW, Robertson JFR, Blamey RW, Nicholson RI: Ki67 immunostaining in primary breast cancer: pathological and clinical associations. Br J Cancer 1989 (59): 943-947

91 Hug V, Thames H, Bentzen S: Predictors of hormone response for patients with ER-unknown breast tumors. Br J Cancer 1989 (59): 421-425

92 Sacannijotti G, Bonadonna G: The pathologist and the clinical oncologist: a new effective partnership in assessing tumor prognosis. Eur J Cancer Clin Oncol 1989 (25): 585-598

# Prognostic Factors in Node-Negative Breast Cancer Patients

Ingegerd Balslev [1,3], Karin Zedeler [2], Susan M. Thorpe [3], Birgitte Bruun Rasmussen [4], and Henning T. Mouridsen [1]

1 Department of Oncology, Rigshospitalet, Copenhagen, Denmark
2 Danish Breast Cancer Cooperative Group (DBCG), The Finsen Institute/Rigshospitalet, Copenhagen, Denmark
3 Department of Tumour Endocrinology, The Fibiger Institute, The Danish Cancer Society, Copenhagen, Denmark
4 Department of Pathology, Roskilde County Hospital, Denmark

The decision to offer adjuvant systemic therapy to a patient with primary breast cancer depends on the expected benefit in terms of improved recurrence-free survival and overall survival in relation to the expected harm in terms of side effects, socioeconomic costs, and possible overtreatment.

The benefits have been extensively analysed in overviews by the Early Breast Cancer Trialists Collaborative Group [1]. A significant proportional reduction in mortality (26% ± 7%) has been demonstrated in patients <50 years old who received multiple-agent chemotherapy, and a reduction of similar order of magnitude (20% ± 3%) has been achieved in patients ≥50 years of age, treated with tamoxifen.

The vast majority of the patients included in these overview analyses were node positive, but retrospective overview analyses of subgroups indicate that the proportional reduction in mortality is similar in the node-positive and node-negative patients [2]. However, it should be emphasised that these retrospective analyses may be biased, due to variability in reporting techniques, definitions, methodologies and statistics [3]. On the other hand, recently published prospective trials in node-negative patients confirm the data from the retrospective subgroup analysis [4-7].

From trials as those cited above, it is possible to estimate the absolute benefit of adjuvant therapy, which is expressed by the number of patients who are cured with the therapy, and the disadvantage of therapy, which is expressed as the sum of those patients who die in spite of therapy plus those who would have been alive without the adjuvant therapy [8]. It is apparent from such analyses that the problem of overtreatment becomes more pronounced the better the prognosis of the treated patient group is.

In the Western world, approximately 150,000 node-negative breast cancer patients are identified annually. Thirty percent of these patients, i.e., 50,000, will ultimately die from their disease. If the proportional reduction of mortality with adjuvant systemic therapy is taken to be 20%, the number of deaths could be reduced to 40,000. However, saving the lives of these 10,000 women requires treatment of 150,000, an overtreatment of 140,000 individuals. Of the overtreated patients, 40,000 will die of their disease in spite of treatment, while 100,000 will have the same survival as they would have had without treatment.

## Prognostic and Predictive Factors

From these data it is obviously very important to discover ways in which patients can be selected according to their prognosis (i.e., by defining significant prognostic factors) and to select patients for treatment according to the probability of their responding to that specific therapy (i.e., by defining predictive factors).

Little is known about the predictive value of different characteristics of the primary tumour. Conflicting data have been reported even for such an extensively studied factor as oestro-

gen receptor (ER) status. These discrepancies have been reviewed elsewhere [3,8].
This chapter will be focussed on the description of the prognostic value of clinical, histopathological, biochemical and proliferative features of primary node-negative breast cancer. The presentation will be divided into 2 parts. First, data for the classical prognostic factors will be presented based upon the trials conducted by the Danish Breast Cancer Cooperative Group, and second, some new factors of possible prognostic value will be reviewed. The latter is not intended to be an extensive survey of all possible prognostic factors, but discusses some more recent studies that reflect the present areas of research.

## Classical Prognostic Factors Illustrated by the DBCG Protocols for Low-Risk Patients

The Danish Breast Cancer Cooperative Group (DBCG) was established in 1976. The structure of the organisation and the project have been described elsewhere [9].
The DBCG programme for low-risk patients comprises 2 protocols, DBCG 77-a and DBCG 82-a (recruitment from 1977 to 1982 and from 1982, respectively). In both protocols, low risk is defined as absence of tumour-positive nodes in the axilla, size of tumour less than 5 cm in diameter, and no histological evidence of invasion to skin or deep fascia. In the DBCG 82-a protocol, a further criterion is that only patients <70 years are included. In order to have comparable results from the 2 protocols, patients from the DBCG 77-a protocol ≥70 years old are excluded in the following.
The DBCG register has information about a number of prognostic variables for each patient, so it is possible to evaluate the importance of each of these variables. The classical prognostic variables are: age of the patient, menopausal status, size of the primary tumour, number of lymph nodes removed, histological grade and ER- and progesterone receptor (PgR) status.
It turned out that the prognosis for the low-risk patients was almost identical in the 77 and 82 protocols. This implies that the patients in the 2 protocols may be considered together in the evaluation of most of the prognostic variables. The only exception is tumour size, which was graded by the surgeon in the 77 protocol, while the grading in the 82 protocol was performed by the pathologist. Some data are not available for all patients. Thus, the histological grading is relevant for ductal carcinomas only and determination of receptor values was not started until 1980 and has not been carried out for all patients.
The importance of receptor value is related to menopausal status [10]. Therefore, the values for the receptor variables have been divided into pre- and postmenopausal patients. 2405 patients entered the DBCG 77-a protocol, while by September 1, 1989, 4648 patients were registered in the DBCG 82-a protocol. Thus, there is a total of 7053 patients in the 2 low-risk protocols.
The value of these prognostic variables can be evaluated separately for each variable. This evaluation may be founded on either time to recurrence or time to death. Since the purpose is to estimate the primary prognostic importance of the variables, time to recurrence is the more appropriate event. After recurrence, the patients receive different systemic therapies that alter the course of the disease.
The prognostic variables by univariate analyses in the DBCG protocols are shown in Table 1, together with p-values for the life-table curves for recurrence-free survival (RFS). Nearly all prognostic variables significantly influence the prognosis when considered separately.
As many of the prognostic factors are significantly correlated to each other, it becomes an essential problem to identify those prognostic factors that act independently. It has been argued elsewhere [11] that such questions can only be properly addressed by more complex statistical models, such as the Cox regression model for survival data [12]. In the Cox model, several prognostic variables may be handled at the same time in order to determine their relative importance. In the model for survival data, the hazard (intensity) of recurrence or death for a given patient is the product of a function of time since mastectomy and a term describing the effect of the prognostic vari-

ables. The general formulation of the model is:

$$\lambda(t;\underline{z}) = \lambda_o(t) \exp(\beta_1 z_1 + \ldots + \beta_K z_K)$$

where t denotes time since mastectomy and z = $(z_1,\ldots,z_K)$ the values of the prognostic variables; $\beta_1,\ldots,\beta_K$ are unknown regression coefficients to be estimated, describing the influence of the corresponding prognostic variables $z_1,\ldots, z_K$. Finally, $\lambda_o(t)$ represents the baseline hazard, i.e., the hazard for a patient at time t after mastectomy for whom $z_1 = z_2 = \ldots z_K = 0$.

The regression coefficients $\beta_1,\ldots, \beta_K$ can be estimated by maximising the partial likelihood function [12]. Hypothesis tests are based on the partial likelihood ratio statistic -2 log Q, which is approximately chi-square distributed with degrees of freedom equal to the reduction in numbers of parameters.

A basic assumption underlying the regression model is that the effect of the prognostic factors is time-independent and multiplicative. These assumptions must be checked for each factor by stratifying according to levels of the factor and verifying whether the underlying intensities estimated are proportional.

**Table 1.** Prognostic variables in protocols DBCG 77-a and 82-a. Univariate analyses

| Prognostic variable | Number of patients Total | Group | | | p-value Lifetable analysis |
|---|---|---|---|---|---|
| | | pre- | post- | | |
| Menopausal status | 7039 | 3433 | 3606 | | 0.46 |
| Age, premenopausal | | < 40 | 40-49 | ≥ 50 | |
| | 3433 | 665 | 1890 | 878 | 0.0001 |
| Age, postmenopausal | | < 50 | 50-59 | 60-69 | |
| | 3606 | 54 | 1295 | 2257 | 0.08 |
| Tumour size, mm | | 0-9 | 10-19 | 20-49 | |
| DBCG 77-a | 2172 | 31 | 314 | 1827 | < 0.0001 |
| DBCG 82-a | 4498 | 503 | 1911 | 2084 | < 0.0001 |
| Removed lymph nodes | | 1-2 | 3-4 | ≥ 5 | |
| | 6825 | 928 | 1595 | 4302 | 0.0001 |
| Histological grade | | I | II | III | |
| | 5422 | 2069 | 2570 | 783 | < 0.0001 |
| Oestrogen receptor | | 0-9 | ≥ 10 | | |
| Premenopausal | 688 | 223 | 465 | | 0.01 |
| Postmenopausal | 983 | 198 | 785 | | 0.56 |
| Progesterone receptor | | 0-9 | ≥ 10 | | |
| Premenopausal | 632 | 182 | 450 | | 0.0005 |
| Postmenopausal | 747 | 260 | 487 | | 0.79 |

In the multivariate analysis, the scoring of the prognostic values is essential and may give rise to substantial problems of interpretation of the results, especially when variables are scored in 3 levels as previously discussed [11].

A detailed multivariate analysis of the DBCG 82-a data requires prolonged clinical follow-up. Consequently, this review will be limited to the presentation of previously published data from the DBCG material.

The study by Rank et al. [13] analysed data from the DBCG 77-a low-risk protocol. The classical prognostic variables, with the exception of receptor status, were included in their Cox analysis and they concluded that tumour size, number of removed nodes and nuclear pleomorphism were the most important prognostic factors. The other components used for histological grading, i.e., the number of mitoses and tubule formation, did not significantly contribute to the prognostic characterisation. Likewise, the histological grade as such did not contribute to prognosis when considered in the multivariate analysis at the same time as the nuclear pleomorphism.

Another study, which encompassed a subset of patients from the DBCG 77 and the DBCG 82 low-risk protocols, included receptor status in the Cox analysis [14]. For histological grading, this study based itself on the data from Rank et al. [13], and included only pleomorphism in the multivariate analysis. Again, the pleomorphism was observed to be the only significant prognostic variable, while the value of the PgR status approached significance. However, when Zedeler [11] applied the Cox analysis to the DBCG 82 material, overall histological grade was observed to be the chief prognostic tool, mainly because of the variables mitoses and tubule formation. The reason for this discrepancy is not quite clear. One explanation might be that the histological grade as originally published by Bloom and Richardson [15] was never intended to be considered as single entities (mitosis, nuclear pleomorphism, tubule formation) and when doing this, one may be faced with the classical statistical problem of mass significance.

The conclusion from these studies is that the grade, or single components thereof, seems to be the most important of the well-established prognostic factors for primary tumours. Similar conclusions have been drawn by other authors [16-18]. However, the reproducibility has been questioned by some authors [19-21] but has been shown to be excellent if proper measures are taken to standardise the methodology [18,21].

Future studies should carefully reanalyse the reproducibility of the grading and also reanalyse the relative prognostic role of the single components of the grading as emphasised by the results from the Danish analyses [11,13]. From the data available, it can be concluded that the grading should be included in the Cox analysis when evaluating the value of the new, more sophisticated and expensive, methods.

## New Factors of Possible Prognostic Value

The ongoing research for new and more powerful prognostic variables in breast cancer has provided us with many new candidates. When evaluating these candidates in the node-negative subgroup, we are faced with 2 major problems. Firstly, a multivariate Cox regression analysis including the classical prognostic factors, especially those which are thought to express the same biological property as the new one, must be performed in order to evaluate whether the new factor contains independent prognostic information. Secondly, most of the published studies concerning prognostic variables include in the Cox analysis node-positive patients, who have received adjuvant therapy. A separate evaluation of the non-treated node-negative subgroup is then impossible, and such an evaluation is necessary since the significant prognostic indicators in node-negative patients are not the same as for the node-positive patients or for the population in general. One reason for this could be that the tumours of the node-negative patients are in an earlier biological stage, and the indicators of tumour progression may therefore differ from those of tumours at a later stage. Another reason could be that the prognostic variables in patient populations which include treated patients contain an element of prediction, i.e., the prognostic variables are influenced by the effect of the treatment. An example could be that tumours with a high proliferative rate have a poor prognosis when untreated, but they are at the same time the most responsive to chemotherapy. So, when treated, the negative effect of the high proliferative rate will be balanced or even outweighed by the positive treatment effect. This phenomenon may also be the reason why the prognostic variables within the untreated node-negative group differ according to the endpoint, i.e., survival or RFS, since the effect of post-recurrence treatment is included in survival analysis but not in RFS analysis.

### *Thymidine Labelling Index*

Many of the investigations on prognostic variables focus on factors which express the proliferative potential of the tumour. One of these is the thymidine labelling index (TLI). In this technique, fresh tumour specimens are incubated with tritiated thymidine. The radioactive DNA-precursor is incorporated in the DNA synthesising cells and autoradiography makes it possible to visualise and count the number of labelled tumour cells. Numerous clinical studies have been performed in solid tumours, including breast cancer, and they have proved its prognostic value mostly by univariate analysis [22]. Only few papers deal with node-negative patients and contain multivariate analysis including histological grade. Multivariate studies concerning either exclusively node-negative patients or including histological grade or PgR status in the Cox analysis are reviewed in Table 2. It appears that the histological grade may play an important role in predicting both survival and RFS. Furthermore, the ER status seems to be important in predicting survival but not recurrence, possibly due to a high degree of antihormone-responsiveness in the ER-positive group. The data emphasise the importance of including all classical prognostic factors and distinguishing between survival and RFS. Especially in the case of the thymidine labelling index, it is important to include histological grade since it contains a score for mitotic activity which may, to some extent, express the same tumour characteristics as the thymidine labelling index. Moreover, thymidine labelling is a tedious and time-consuming procedure compared to grading.

**Table 2.** Multivariate studies of thymidine labelling index (TLI) in primary breast cancer

| Reference | No.pts. | Stage/ node-status | Adj. syst. therapy | Follow-up (years) | Additonal variables tested | Independent variables with endpoint RFS | Independent variables with endpoint Survival |
|---|---|---|---|---|---|---|---|
| Tubiana et al. [23] | 96 | stage 1-3b | none | 15 | no.pos.ln [a] | grade<br>TLI | grade<br>TLI<br>size [b] |
| Meyer et al. [24] | 414 | stage 1-3 | some | 5 | PgR | size<br>no.pos.ln<br>TLI | size<br>TLI<br>no.pos.ln<br>ER |
| Silvestrini et al. [25] | 354 | node neg. | none | 6 | | TLI<br>size | TLI<br>ER |
| Courdi et al. [26] | 142 | node neg. | none | 8 | size<br>grade<br>ER<br>PgR | TLI<br>PgR[b] | not estimated |

a number of positive lymph nodes; b marginally significant

**Table 3.** Multivariate studies of the prognostic value of DNA content in primary breast cancer

| Reference | No. pts. | Stage/ node-status | Adj.syst. therapy | Follow-up (years) | Material/ method | Additional variables tested | Independent variables with endpoint RFS | survival |
|---|---|---|---|---|---|---|---|---|
| Klintenberg et al. [31] | 210 | stage 1-3 | some | 5 | frozen FCM and static | | stage nodal status SPF ER | |
| Dowle et al. [27] | 348 | stage 1-3 | none | 7.5 | paraffin FCM | ploidy ER (?) | | nodal status grade status |
| Cornelisse et al. [32] | 353 | stage 1-3 | some | 7 | frozen/ paraffin FCM | | nodal status size ploidy [a] | nodal status ER ploidy [b] |
| Fallenius et al. [28] | 227 | stage 1-3 | none | 10 | fixed aspiration static | grade stage | | histogram type (Auer), nodal status, size |
| Fallenius et al. [28] | 129 | node neg. | none | 10 | fixed aspiration static | size,grade ER, PgR | histogram type (Auer), others not mentioned | |
| Kallionemi et al. [33] | 297 | stage 1-3 | some | 8 | paraffin FCM | ER | | histogram type (comb.ploidy/ SPF) size, PgR nodal status |
| von Rosen et al. [34] | 464 | stage 1-3 | some | 3 | frozen aspiration static | ER | size, nodal status histogram type (Auer) | |
| von Rosen et al. [34] | 294 | node neg. | none (?) | 3 | frozen aspiration static | ER | histogram type (Auer) size | |
| Clark et al. [30] | 345 | node neg. | some | 7 | frozen powders/ FCM | ER SPF | ploidy [b] | PgR |
| Muss et al. [29] | 101 | node neg. | none | 9 | frozen pieces FCM | ploidy [b] ER PgR | *neither* ploidy *nor* SPF | % S + % G2/M ER [a] |

a marginally significant; b diploid versus aneuploid

### *DNA Ploidy and S-Phase Fraction*

A DNA histogram, i.e., a distribution of the number of cells with a specific DNA content, can be obtained either by static cytophotometry or by flow cytometry (FCM). The DNA index (DI) or ploidy is the DNA content of the GI tumour cells in relation to the DNA content of normal diploid cells. The fraction of cells in S-phase, i.e., DNA synthesis phase, is estimated from the histogram by various mathematical methods.

Numerous investigations have demonstrated the prognostic value of DNA ploidy and S-phase fraction (SPF). Only few authors, however, include Cox analysis with histological

grade. Nuclear or histological grading is presumably important, since tumour ploidy and S-phase fraction may reflect nuclear pleomorphism and mitotic activity, respectively. This point of view is supported by the fact that several authors have found that ploidy and histological grade are correlated [27-29].
Two recent studies have restricted themselves to node-negative patients. Clark et al. [30] investigated 395 breast cancer specimens and obtained useable histograms from 345 (87%). In a Cox model, which did not include histological grading, they found that ploidy was the only significant prognostic indicator using RFS as endpoint, while PgR status was the only significant indicator using survival as endpoint. Furthermore, a multivariate analysis of the diploid group showed the S-phase fraction (SPF) to be the only significant factor with respect to both RFS and survival. In the aneuploid group, SPF was not significant, probably due to overlapping S-phases interfering with the precise mathematical estimation of the S-phase. Muss et al. [29] analysed the DNA content of 101 tumours from untreated patients and found in a multivariate analysis in which grading was not included that the number of cells in S-phase plus G2/M-phase was an independent prognostic factor with respect to survival, while the DNA index was of no significance. A number of important studies are summarised in Table 3.
In conclusion, the value of DNA content as an independent prognostic factor in untreated node-negative patients has, as yet, not been fully clarified. For this purpose, standardisation with respect to patient material, technique and histogram interpretation is highly needed.

## *Ki-67 Growth Fraction*

The ideal cell kinetic parameter remains to be found. A more recent approach is estimation of the growth fraction (GF) by means of the monoclonal antibody Ki-67, which binds to a nuclear antigen expressed exclusively in continously cycling cells and therefore absent in the resting G0 cells [35,36]. The fraction of Ki-67 positive nuclei is measured by immunostaining of fresh frozen tissue sections. Correlations between the Ki-67 growth fraction and histological grade and ER content have been found by several groups (Table 4). Whether Ki-67 growth fraction is an independent prognostic factor or even a prognostic factor by univariate analysis remains to be proven. This may take years, since the need for fresh tumour tissue usually implies prospective studies, and in the node-negative patients the recurrence and death rates are low.

**Table 4.** Expression of the Ki-67 antigen in primary breast cancer

| Ref. | No.pts. | Range of Ki-67 positivity | Positive correlation to poor grade | ER- |
|---|---|---|---|---|
| Lellé et al. [37] | 145 | 1-48% | yes | NI [a] |
| McGurrin et al. [38] | 33 | 3-60% | yes | yes |
| Walker et al. [39] | 95 | 0-60% | yes | NI |
| Wrba et al. [40] | 107 | 0.9-26.4% | yes | yes |

a Not investigated

## *Oncogene Expression and Amplification*

Oncogene amplification, i.e., number of gene copies, and expression, i.e., RNA or oncoprotein concentration, as prognostic factors have been studied extensively in recent years. Especially the c-erbB-2 or HER-2/neu oncogene, which is amplified in 25-30% of the tumours, has been investigated in breast cancer. The oncogene amplification is measured by Southern or DNA dot blot analysis, RNA is measured by Northern blot analysis, and the oncoprotein by either Western blot analysis or by immunostaining of histological slides by means of the polyclonal antiserum 21N [41] or by monoclonal antibodies [42]. The latter method can be performed in paraffin-embedded tissue and is consequently applicable in retrospective studies. A correlation between gene amplification and oncoprotein expression measured by the immuno-

**Table 5.** Multivariate studies of the c-erbB-2 or HER-2/neu oncogene in primary breast cancer

| Reference | No. pts. | Stage/ node-status | Method | Pos. (%) | Additional variables tested | Independent variables with endpoint RFS | survival |
|---|---|---|---|---|---|---|---|
| Tandon et al. [45] | 350 | node pos. | expression Western | 17 | ER | no.pos.ln. HER-2/neu size PgR [b] | no.pos.ln. PgR HER-2/neu size |
| Slamon et al. [46] | 86 | node pos. | amplification Southern | 40 | size ER PgR | no.pos.ln. [a] HER-2/neu | no.pos.ln. HER-2/neu |
| Wright et al. [47] | 102 | stage 1-3 | expression polyclonal 21N | 58 | grade ER EGFR | nodal status 21N-staining size | nodal status 21N-staining |
| Slamon et al. [48] | 345 | node pos. | amplification Southern | 27 | size ER PgR | no.pos.ln. HER-2/neu | no.pos.ln. HER-2/neu |
| Slamon et al. [48] | 181 | node neg. | amplification Southern | 25 | size ER PgR | *not* HER-2/neu | *not* HER-2/neu |
| Tsuda et al. [49] | 176 | stage 1-4 | amplification Slot-blot c-myc | 16 4 | size | no.pos.ln. c-erbB-2 c-myc | no.pos.ln. c-erbB-2 |
| Walker et al. [50] | 85 | stage 1-4 | expression polyclonal 21N | 24 | nodal status stage grade | 21N-staining others not given | 21N-staining others not given |

a number of positive lymph nodes; b marginally significant

staining technique [43,44], and by Western blot analysis [45] has been demonstrated. Seven multivariate studies, all but one including node-positive patients, are summarised in Table 5. Table 6 lists the results of 6 univariate studies, 5 of which including exclusively node-negative patients. In conclusion, amplification or expression of the c-erbB-2 oncogene is evidently an independent prognostic factor in node-positive but not in node-negative primary breast cancer. This very fact indicates the need for investigations on prognostic variables solely in the node-negative subgroup.

Many other oncogenes and co-amplifications, like c-myc, which codes for a nuclear protein regulating gene expression and int-2/hst-1, which codes for a fibroblast growth factor, have been investigated in breast cancer, but their prognostic value is not established.

Several oncoproteins are growth factor receptors. Thus, the c-erbB-1 oncogene codes for the epithelial growth factor receptor (EGFR), and the c-erbB-2 oncoprotein has high homology with the EGF-receptor. The growth factor receptors may well prove to be useful prognostic factors as reviewed by Klijn and Foekens elsewhere in this monograph.

## *The $M_r$ 52,000 Cathepsin D Protease*

An attempt to assay the metastatic potential of the tumours has been performed by Thorpe et al. [52] in DBCG patients. This was done by measuring the protease $M_r$ 52,000 cathepsin D, which can degrade extracellular matrices and proteoglycans and is induced by oestrogens in ER-positive breast cancer cell lines [53]. The concentration of the total cathepsin

**Table 6.** Univariate studies of the c-erbB-2 or HER-2/neu oncogene in node-negative breast cancer

| Reference | No. pts. | Method | Pos. (%) | Univariate significance RFS | survival |
|---|---|---|---|---|---|
| van de Vijver et al. [42] | 189 [a] | expression, monoclonal 9G6 | 14 | no | yes |
| Tandon et al. [45] | 378 | expression, Western | | no | no |
| Wright et al. [47] | 44 | expression, polyclonal 21N | | no | yes |
| Slamon et al. [48] | 181 | amplification, Southern | 25 | no | no |
| Tsuda et al. [49] | 73 | amplification, Slot-blot | | no | no |
| Ro et al. [51] | 66 | amplification, Southern/ dot blot | 20 | no | yes |

a) stage II, 58% node-negative

D was assayed in cytosols from 396 primary breast cancers, 203 (51%) of which were node negative. Patients with high cathepsin D concentrations had shorter recurrence-free survival and a trend toward shorter overall survival. In the multivariate analysis including histological grade, cathepsin D status together with number of tumour-positive lymph nodes and tumour size were found to be independent prognostic factors for recurrence-free survival in the pre-/perimenopausal as well as the postmenopausal women. Multivariate analysis was not performed separately in node-negative patients, but univariate analysis showed cathepsin D status to be of prognostic value in this subgroup.

## Conclusion

The introduction of adjuvant systemic therapy to node-negative patients makes the development of methods to improve the prognostic characterisation of the individual patient particularly urgent.

From this brief review, it seems that, among the classical factors, histological grade is a strong prognostic variable, if proper measures are taken to improve the reproducibility as exemplified by the DBCG studies.

Over the past 10 years, we have witnessed the development of new methods focussing on factors that express the proliferative potential of the tumour. Some of these variables do seem to predict the prognosis of the patients but the available data are conflicting and call for carefully conducted quality-control studies to analyse intra- and interlaboratory variation. In the evaluation of the ultimate value of these methods, the multivariate analyses should include at least the more easily available histological grading and steroid receptor status of the tumour.

## Acknowledgement

Ingegerd Balslev is sponsored by The Danish Medical Research Council, The Arvid Nilsson Foundation and the Max Fodgaard Foundation.

## REFERENCES

1 Early Breast Cancer Triallists Collaborative Group: Effects of adjuvant tamoxifen and of cytotoxic therapy on mortality in early breast cancer. An overview of 61 randomized trials among 28,896 women. New Engl J Med 1988 (319): 1681-1692
2 Early Breast Cancer Triallists Collaborative Group. 1989, in preparation
3 Mouridsen HT, Rose C: Attempting to understand differences between the results of the main trials of adjuvant tamoxifen in primary breast cancer. In: Bresciani F, King RJB, Lippman ME (eds) Progress in Cancer Research and Treatment Vol 35: Hormones and Cancer 3. Raven Press, New York 1988, pp 417-422
4 Fisher B, Redmond C, Dimitrov NV et al: A randomized clinical trial evaluating sequential methotrexate and fluorouracil in the treatment of patients with node-negative breast cancer who have estrogen-receptor-negative tumors. N Engl J Med 1989 (320):473-478
5 Fisher B, Constantino J, Redmond C et al: A randomized clinical trial evaluating tamoxifen in the treatment of patients with node-negative breast cancer who have estrogen-receptor-positive tumors. N Engl J Med 1989 (320): 479-484
6 Mansour EG, Gray R, Shatila AH et al: Efficacy of adjuvant chemotherapy in high-risk node-negative breast cancer: an intergroup study. N Engl J Med 1989 (320): 485-490
7 The Ludwig Breast Cancer Study Group: Prolonged disease-free survival after one course of perioperative adjuvant chemotherapy for node-negative breast cancer. N Engl J Med 1989 (320):491-496
8 Mouridsen HT: Adjuvant hormonal therapy: Whom to treat. Horm Res l989 (32, Suppl 1):169-172
9 Andersen KW and Mouridsen HT: Danish Breast Cancer Cooperative Group (DBCG). A description of the register of the nation-wide programme for primary breast cancer. Acta Oncologica 1988 (27):627-647
10 Thorpe SM, Rose C, Pedersen BV and Rasmussen BB: Estrogen and progesterone receptor profile patterns in primary breast cancer. Breast Cancer Res Treat 1983 (3):103-110
11 Zedeler K: Assessment and presentation of survival experience in the Danish Breast Cancer Cooperative Group. Acta Oncologica 1988 (27):649-662
12 Cox DR: Regression models and life tables (with discussion). J R Stat Soc B 1972 (34):187-202
13 Rank F, Dombernowsky P, Jespersen NCB et al: Histologic malignancy grading of invasive ductal breast carcinoma. Cancer 1987 (60):1299-1305
14 Thorpe SM, Rose C, Rasmussen BB et al: Prognostic value of steroid hormone receptors: Multivariate analysis of systemically untreated patients with node-negative primary breast cancer. Cancer Res 1987 (47):6126-6133
15 Bloom HJ and Richardson WW: Histological grading and prognosis in breast cancer. Br J Cancer 1957 (11):359-377
16 le Doussal V, Tubiana-Hulin M, Friedman S et al: Prognostic value of histologic grade nuclear components of Scarff-Bloom-Richardson (SBR). Cancer 1989 (64): 1914-1921
17 Fisher ER: Prognostic and therapeutic significance of pathological features of breast cancer. NCI Monogr 1986 (1):29-34
18 Contesso G, Mouriesse H, Friedman S et al: The importance of histologic grade in long-term prognosis of breast cancer: A study of 1010 patients, uniformly treated at the Institut Gustave Roussy. J Clin Oncol 1987 (5):1378-1386
19 Stenkvist B, Bengtsson E, Eriksson O et al: Histopathological systems of breast cancer classification. Reproducibility and clinical significance. J Clin Pathol 1983 (36):392-398
20 Davies BW, Gelber D, Goldhirsch A et al: Prognostic significance of tumor grade in clinical trials of adjuvant therapy for breast cancer with axillary lymph nodes metastasis. Cancer 1986 (58):2662-2670
21 Jacquemier J, Vague D, Lieutaud R et al: Definition et reproductibilite du grading de Scarff et Bloom. In: Evaluation des mouens de diagnostic du cancer du sein. IIle Journees de la Societe Francaise du Senologie et de Pathologie Mammaire. Versailles. JMT Conseil 1981 pp 173-185
22 Tubiana M and Courdi A: Cell proliferation kinetics in human solid tumors: relation to probability of metastatic dissemination and long-term survival. Radiother Oncol 1989 (15):1-18
23 Tubiana M, Pejovic MH, Chavaudra N et al: The long-term prognostic significance of the thymidine labelling index in breast cancer. Int J Cancer 1984 (33):441-445
24 Meyer JS and Province M: Proliferative index of breast carcinoma by thymidine labeling: prognostic power independent of stage, estrogen and progesterone receptors. Breast Cancer Res Treat 1988 (12):191-204
25 Silvestrini R, Daidone MG, Valagussa P et al: Cell kinetics as a prognostic indicator in node-negative breast cancer. Eur J Cancer Clin Oncol 1989 (25):1165-1171
26 Courdi A, Héry M, Dahan E et al: Factors affecting relapse in node-negative breast cancer. A multivariate analysis including the labeling index. Eur J Cancer Clin Oncol 1989 (25):351-356
27 Dowle CS, Owainati A, Robins A et al: Prognostic significance of the DNA content of human breast cancer. Br J Surg 1987 (74):133-136
28 Fallenius AG, Franzen SA, Auer GU: Predictive value of nuclear DNA content in breast cancer in relation to clinical and morphologic factors. Cancer 1988 (62):521-530
29 Muss HB, Kute TE, Case LD et al: The relation of flow cytometry to clinical and biologic characteristics in women with node negative primary breast cancer. Cancer 1989 (64):1894-1900
30 Clark GM, Dressler LG, Owens MA et al: Prediction of relapse or survival in patients with node-negative breast cancer by DNA flow cytometry. N Engl J Med 1989 (320):627-633
31 Klintenberg C, Stål O, Nordenskjöld B et al: Proliferative index, cytosol estrogen receptor and

axillary node status as prognostic predictors in human mammary carcinoma. Breast Cancer Res Treat 1986 (7):99-106
32 Cornelisse CJ, van de Velde CJH, Caspers RJC et al: DNA ploidy and survival in breast cancer patients. Cytometry 1987 (8):225-234
33 Kallioniemi OP, Blanco G, Alavaikko M et al: Improving the prognostic value of DNA flow cytometry in breast cancer by combining DNA index and S-phase fraction. Cancer 1988 (62):2183-2190
34 von Rosen A, Rutqvist LE, Carstensen J et al: Prognostic value of nuclear DNA content in broast cancer in relation to tumor size, nodal status and estrogen receptor content. Breast Cancer Res Treat 1989 (13):23-32
35 Gerdes J, Schwab U, Lemke H and Stein H: Production of a mouse monoclonal antibody reactive with a human nuclear antigen associated with cell proliferation. Int J Cancer 1983 (31):13-20
36 Gerdes J, Lemke H, Baisch H et al: Cell cycle analysis of a cell proliferation-associated human nuclear antigen defined by the monoclonal antibody Ki-67. J Immunol 1984 (133):1710-1715
37 Lellé RJ, Heidenreich W, Stauch G and Gerdes J: The correlation of growth fractions with histologic grading and lymph node status in human mammary carcinoma. Cancer 1987 (59):83-88
38 McGurrin JF, Doria MI, Dawson PJ et al: Assessment of tumor cell kinetics by immunohistochemistry in carcinoma of breast. Cancer 1987 (59):1744-1750
39 Walker RA and Camplejohn RS: Comparison of monoclonal antibody Ki-67 reactivity with grade and DNA flow cytometry of breast carcinomas. Br J Cancer 1988 (57):281-283
40 Wrba F, Chott A, Reiner A et al: Ki-67 immunoreactivity in breast carcinomas in relation to transferrin receptor expression, estrogen receptor status and morphological criteria. Oncology 1989 (46):255-259
41 Gullick WJ, Berger MS, Bennett PLP et al: Expression of the c-erbB-2 protein in normal and transformed cell. Int J Cancer 1987 (40):246-254
42 van de Vijver MJ, Peterse JL, Mooi WJ et al. Neu-protein overexpression in breast cancer. Association with comedo-type ductal carcinoma in situ and limited prognostic value in Stage II breast cancer. N Engl J Med 1988 (319): 1239-1245
43 Venter DJ, Tuzi NL, Kumar S and Gullick WJ: Overexpression of the c-erbB-2 oncoprotein in human breast carcinomas: Immunohistological assessment correlates with gene amplification. Lancet I987 (ii):69-72
44 Berger MS, Locher GW, Saurer S et al: Correlation of c-erbB-2 gene amplification and protein expression in human breast carcinoma with nodal status and nuclear grading. Cancer Res 1988 (48):1238-1243
45 Tandon AK, Clark GM, Chamness GC et al: HER-2/neu oncogene protein and prognosis in breast cancer. J Clin Oncol 1989 (7): 1120-1128
46 Slamon DJ, Clark GM, Wong SG et al: Human breast cancer: Correlation of relapse and survival with amplification of the HER-2/neu oncogene. Science 1987 (235):177-182
47 Wright C, Angus B, Nicholson S et al: Expression of c-erbB-2 oncoprotein: A prognostic indicator in human breast cancer. Cancer Res 1989 (49):2087-2090
48 Slamon DJ, Godolphin W, Jones LA et al: Studies of the HER-2/neu proto-oncogene in human breast and ovarian cancer. Science 1989 (244):707-712
49 Tsuda H, Hirohashi S, Shimosato Y et al: Correlation between long-term survival in breast cancer patients and amplification of two putative oncogene-coamplification units: hst-1/int-2 and c-erbB-2/ear-1. Cancer Res 1989 (49):3104-3108
50 Walker RA, Gullick WJ, Varley JM: An evaluation of immunoreactivity for c-erbB-2 protein as a marker of poor short-term prognosis in breast cancer. Br J Cancer 1989 (60):426-429
51 Ro J, El-Naggar A, Ro JY et al: c-erbB-2 amplification in node-negative human breast cancer. Cancer Res 1989 (49):6941-6944
52 Thorpe SM, Rochefort H, Garcia M et al: Association between high concentrations of $M_r$ 52,000 cathepsin D and poor prognosis in primary human breast cancer. Cancer Res 1989 (49): 6008-6014
53 Vignon F, Capony F, Chambon M et al: Autocrine growth stimulation of the MCF-7 breast cancer cells by the estrogen-stimulated 52K protein. Endocrinology 1986 (118):1537-1545

# Long-Term Tamoxifen Therapy: An Appropriate Chemosuppressive Treatment for Breast Cancer

V. Craig Jordan

Department of Human Oncology, University of Wisconsin Clinical Cancer Center, Madison, WI 53792, U.S.A.

Tamoxifen (Nolvadex®) is a non-steroidal antioestrogen and the first-line endocrine therapy for breast cancer [1-3]. The drug has proved to have efficacy as an adjuvant in node-positive disease [3,4] and increasing numbers of node-negative breast cancer patients are being treated with tamoxifen [5]. A remarkable feature of treatment with tamoxifen is the low incidence of side effects [1,3]. These clinical observations and the large body of evidence from the laboratory [6,7] have focussed clinical attention on long-term, or indefinite (treatment until relapse), adjuvant tamoxifen therapy [5,8-10].

To date, no generally reported major side effects have been observed that should restrict the long-term use of tamoxifen. Fortuitously, tamoxifen seems to possess an appropriate level of oestrogenic action to produce favourable effects upon bone [11,12] and circulating lipids [13]. Therefore, earlier concerns that tamoxifen would provoke osteoporosis or atherosclerosis seem to be unfounded. Nevertheless, further research is required to ensure the safety of tamoxifen and, most importantly, the well-being of the patients. In fact, it may transpire that tamoxifen provides a general improvement in the health of women after the menopause, over and above the ability to save lives, as an agent to suppress the recurrence of breast cancer.

The ubiquitous use of tamoxifen in all stages of breast cancer has provided the oncologist with a safe therapy but it would be naive to suggest that tamoxifen can cure, or indeed, indefinitely control the recurrence of the disease. Drug resistance will almost certainly occur. Concerns about this aspect of treatment retarded the early implementation of long-term adjuvant trials with tamoxifen. The original protocols depended upon 1 or 2 years of treatment [4]. However, the debate about whether to use long-term adjuvant tamoxifen therapy (5 years) after mastectomy, or wait and use the tamoxifen as a first treatment on relapse, has been resolved by the Scottish trial [10]. Early adjuvant tamoxifen therapy confers a survival advantage when compared to a control arm of patients who, in the main, received tamoxifen upon relapse. Premature drug resistance to tamoxifen does not occur during adjuvant therapy. However, it is prudent to consider models for potential drug resistance to develop strategies in the laboratory that, in the decade to come, may be applicable to the clinics.

## Hormone-Responsive Endometrial Carcinoma Growth

Unopposed oestrogen replacement therapy is associated with a low, but significant, incidence of endometrial carcinoma in postmenopausal women [14,15]. This observation should not have been a surprise since earlier reports from the laboratory and clinic had indicated that this action of oestrogen was possible [16]. The medical community responded to the knowledge by integrating progestin treatment to maintain menstrual cycles (through withdrawal bleeding) and to prevent occult endometrial carcinoma cells from becoming invasive tumours. Current opinion has it that the overall value of postmenopausal oestrogen replacement therapy could substantially outweigh consideration of the risk of endometrial carcinoma [16-18]. Unopposed oestrogen is the treatment of choice for the hysterectomised patient and the addition of progestin should be considered carefully because of the deleterious effect on the risk for cardiovascular disease [19] and the possible deleterious action in promoting breast cancer [20]. Overall, the benefits of oestrogen to the general health of women outweigh the perceived risks.

As mentioned previously, tamoxifen has some valuable oestrogen-like qualities that may be beneficial to the overall health of the breast cancer patient. The long treatment schedules (5 or 10 years) being evaluated in patients with node-negative disease make this an important consideration for women. Nevertheless, there is a gap in our knowledge about the action of tamoxifen on the uterus during extended therapy. This is currently not a serious omission as the applied treatment is to suppress the recurrence of a fatal disease, breast cancer. Obviously, it would be inappropriate to deny a patient a beneficial therapy for breast cancer because of a perceived risk in the uterus to facilitate the promotion of endometrial carcinoma.

Tamoxifen has an interesting pharmacological profile with a mix of oestrogenic and antioestrogen actions depending upon the target organ, the species or the duration of therapy [1,21]. Although tamoxifen can stimulate the uterus of laboratory animals, it is only a partial oestrogen and blocks the full expression of oestrogen action produced by oestradiol [22].

Tamoxifen has been used successfully to treat advanced endometrial carcinoma [23,24]. Nevertheless, endometrial cancer can occur during the treatment of breast cancer with tamoxifen [25,26]. This is not too surprising since only a fraction of endometrial carcinoma is hormone-responsive, so the majority of disease would not be expected to be controlled by tamoxifen.

Currently there is evidence from only 1 randomised clinical trial [28] and laboratory studies with hormone-responsive endometrial carcinoma from 2 patients [29-31] to demonstrate that tamoxifen can produce an oestrogenic stimulus to promote sustained endometrial tumour growth.

The questions could therefore be asked, based upon the previous debate with postmenopausal oestrogen replacement therapy: 1) does the risk for endometrial carcinoma with tamoxifen outweigh the benefits, and 2) should tamoxifen be combined with progestins to avoid unopposed endometrial stimulation?

The answer to the first question is straightforward. Tamoxifen has proven efficacy for the treatment of node-positive breast cancer [4]. Fortunately, endometrial carcinoma has a good prognosis so that any suspicious bleeding and confirmatory endometrial histology can result in effective treatment by hysterectomy. However, the fact that breast cancer is a fatal disease, and recurrences are invariably impossible to treat, must be the primary reason to maintain adjuvant tamoxifen therapy. Secondarily, the developing information concerning the beneficial effects of the oestrogen-like properties of tamoxifen on bone and plasma lipids may provide additional benefit for the patient.

The answer to the second question is more speculative. There is only a theoretical advantage of using progestins to avoid the possible promotion of endometrial carcinoma due to the oestrogenic influences of tamoxifen. A combination of tamoxifen and progestin has been shown to be less efficacious for the treatment of advanced breast cancer than tamoxifen alone [32] and there are data from laboratory models of breast cancer that progestins can promote carcinogenesis [33]. Indeed, the effects of tamoxifen can be reversed by pregnancy levels of progesterone in carcinogen-induced rat mammary carcinoma models [34,35]. At present, it may be prudent to avoid the introduction of low-dose progestin therapy with tamoxifen as we are unaware of the effects upon breast tissue. Clearly, there is little advantage to resolving endometrial carcinoma but negating the beneficial action of tamoxifen on the appearance of new primary breast tumours [28] or micrometastatic lesions.

## Tamoxifen-Enhanced Breast Tumour Growth?

The long-term treatment of cancer with therapeutic agents invariably results in the development of drug resistance. The length of response of advanced disease to tamoxifen therapy is about 14 months [1] but no clear picture has, as yet, emerged about drug resistance to adjuvant tamoxifen therapy. As a result, laboratory studies are currently under way to develop models to study drug resistance to tamoxifen. Long-term tamoxifen treatment of athymic (immune-deficient) mice implanted with hormone-responsive MCF-7 breast cancer cells, eventually results in tumour growth despite continuing tamoxifen therapy [36,37]. In fact, the tumours still retain hormone receptors and will regain responsiveness to the inhibitory actions of tamoxifen in cell culture [37,38]. The tumour growth appears to be enhanced by tamoxifen in this animal model and tumour growth stops on removal of the stimulus [39]. However, tumour growth will also occur with oestradiol. Therefore, if this form of resistance to tamoxifen therapy ever occurs within the clinic, then it will be unacceptable to stop tamoxifen therapy without implementing another "antioestrogenic" therapy. In fact, it is possible that such a form of drug resistance to tamoxifen has already been observed in trials that compare the efficacy of tamoxifen with aminoglutethimide in crossover studies. Patients appear to have a higher probability of having a second response to aminoglutethimide after a response to tamoxifen than the reverse [40]. Since the tamoxifen was stopped, once aminoglutethimide was started, it is impossible to establish whether the effect is a withdrawal response to tamoxifen or a suppression of oestrogen biosynthesis that had originally reversed the action of tamoxifen.

Another approach is to initiate a research programme to discover novel antihormonal agents devoid of the oestrogenic properties of tamoxifen. Clearly, this strategy again presents a problem with the long-term toxicological questions of osteoporosis and atherosclerosis that could reduce the probability of pure antioestrogens being used to treat node-negative disease. Nevertheless, novel agents have been discovered which exhibit no oestrogenic activity and appear to act as pure antioestrogens [39,41].

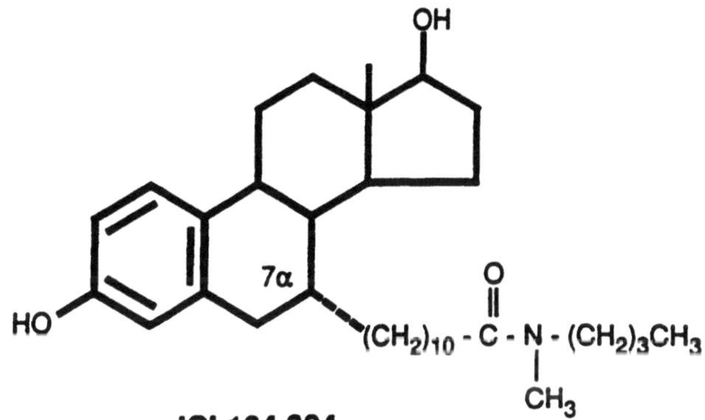


ICI 164,384

Fig. 1.

Although research is at present only being conducted in the laboratory, successful agents may become available for clinical testing in the 1990s. An example of one such compound is illustrated in Figure 1.

## Summary and Conclusions

Tamoxifen is a safe, well-tolerated drug that has proven efficacy in the adjuvant treatment of breast cancer. Concerns about the long-term detrimental effects of an antioestrogen on bone and cardiovascular risk appear to be unfounded and further study may in fact reveal an advantage for tamoxifen-treated women.

Breast cancer is invariably a fatal disease, so clues to successful treatment regimens should be pursued relentlessly. Tamoxifen can increase the survival of breast cancer patients, therefore, perceived risks of developing occult endometrial carcinoma are only of minor concern compared with the certain prognosis of patients denied tamoxifen. Good patient care and regular gynaecological examinations if spotting or bleeding occurs should be the cornerstone of long-term adjuvant tamoxifen therapy.

## REFERENCES

1 Furr BJA, Jordan VC: The pharmacology and clinical uses of tamoxifen. Pharm Ther 1984 (25):127-205
2 Jordan VC (ed) Estrogen/Antiestrogen Action and Breast Cancer Therapy. University of Wisconsin Press, Madison 1986
3 Love RR: Tamoxifen therapy in primary breast cancer: biology, efficacy and side effects. J Clin Oncol 1989 (7):803-815
4 Early Breast Cancer Trialists' Collaborative Group: Effects of adjuvant tamoxifen and of cytotoxic therapy on mortality in early breast cancer. N Engl J Med 1988 (319):1681-1692
5 Fisher B, Costantino J, Redmond C et al: A randomized clinical trial evaluating tamoxifen in the treatment of patients with node negative breast cancer who have estrogen receptor positive tumors. N Engl J Med 1989 (320):479-484
6 Jordan VC: Laboratory studies to develop general principles for the treatment of breast cancer with antiestrogens: problems and potential for future clinical applications. Breast Cancer Res Treat 1983 (3 Suppl):s73-s86
7 Jordan VC: Long-term tamoxifen therapy for breast cancer. In: DeVita VT, Hellman S, Rosenberg S (eds) Important Advances in Oncology. Lippincott, Philadelphia 1989 pp 179-192
8 Tormey DC, Jordan VC: Long-term tamoxifen adjuvant therapy in node-positive breast cancer: a metabolic and pilot clinical study. Breast Cancer Res Treat 1984 (4):297-302
9 Fisher B and other NSABP Investigators: Prolonging tamoxifen for primary breast cancer: findings from the National Surgical Adjuvant Breast and Bowel Project clinical trial. Ann Intern Med 1987 (106):649-654
10 Breast Cancer Trials Committee, Scottish Cancer Trials Office (MRC): Adjuvant tamoxifen in the management of operable breast cancer: the Scottish trial. Lancet 1987 (ii):171-175
11 Love RR, Mazess RB, Tormey DC et al: Bone mineral density in women with breast cancer treated for at least two years with tamoxifen. Breast Cancer Res Treat 1988 (12):297-301
12 Turken S, Siris E, Seldin E et al: Effects of tamoxifen on spinal bone density in women with breast cancer. JNCI 1989 (91):1086-1088
13 Bertelli G, Pronzata P, Amaroso D et al: Adjuvant tamoxifen in primary breast cancer: influence on plasma lipids and antithrombin III levels. Breast Cancer Res Treat 1988 (12):307-310
14 Antunes CM, Stolley PD, Rosenhein NB et al: Endometrial cancer and estrogen use: report of a large case-control study. N Engl J Med 1979 (300):9-13
15 Weiss NS, Szekely DR, Austin DF: Increasing incidence of endometrial cancer in the United States. N Engl J Med 1976 (294):1259-1262
16 Fox H: Endometrial carcinogenesis and its relation to oestrogens. Path Res Pract 1984 (1979):13-19
17 Whithead MI, Fraser D: Controversies concerning the safety of estrogen replacement therapy. Am J Obstet Gynecol 1987 (156):1312-1322
18 Hillner BE, Hollenberg JP, Pauker SG: Postmenopausal estrogen in prevention of osteoporosis. Am J Med 1986 (80):1115-1127
19 Henderson BE, Ross RK, Lobo RA, Pike MC, Mack TM: Re-evaluating the role of progestogen therapy after the menopause. Fert Steril 1988 (498 Suppl):9s-15s
20 Bergkvist L, Adami H-O, Persson I et al: The risk of breast cancer after estrogen and estrogen-progestin replacement. N Engl J Med 1989 (321):293-297
21 Jordan VC, Robinson SP: Species-specific pharmacology of antiestrogens: role of metabolism. Fed Proc 1987 (46):1870-1874
22 Harper MJK, Walpole AL: A new derivative of triphenylethylene: effect on implantation and mode of action in rats. J Reprod Fertil 1967 (13):101-119
23 Broens J, Mouridsen HT, Soerensen HM: Tamoxifen in advanced endometrial carcinoma. Cancer Chemother Pharmacol 1980 (4):805-811
24 Swenerton KD: Treatment of advanced endometrial adenocarcinoma with tamoxifen. Cancer Treat Rep 1980 (64):805-811
25 Killackey MA, Hakes TB, Pierce VK: Endometrial adenocarcinoma in breast cancer patients receiving tamoxifen. Cancer Treat Rep 1985 (69):237-238
26 Hardell L: Tamoxifen as risk factor for carcinoma of corpus uteri. Lancet 1988 (ii):563
27 Hardell L: Pelvic irradiation and tamoxifen as risk factors for carcinoma of corpus uteri. Lancet 1988 (ii):1432
28 Fornander T, Rutqvist LE, Cedermark B et al: Adjuvant tamoxifen in early breast cancer: occurrence of new primary cancers. Lancet 1989 (i):117-120
29 Satyaswaroop PG, Zaino RJ, Mortel R: Estrogen-like effect of tamoxifen on human endometrial carcinoma transplanted into nude mice. Cancer Res 1984 (44):4006-4010
30 Clark CL, Satyaswaroop PG: Photoaffinity labeling of the progesterone receptor from human endometrial carcinoma. Cancer Res 1985 (45):5417-5420
31 Gottardis MM, Robinson SP, Satyaswaroop PG, Jordan VC: Contrasting actions of tamoxifen on endometrial and breast tumor growth in the athymic mouse. Cancer Res 1988 (48):812-815
32 Mouridsen HT, Ellemann K, Mattsson W et al: Therapeutic effect of tamoxifen versus tamoxifen combined with medroxyprogesterone acetate in advanced breast cancer in postmenopausal women. Cancer Treat Rep 1979 (63):171-175
33 Jabara AG, Toyens PH, Harcourt AG: Effects of time and duration of progesterone administration on mammary tumors induced by 7,12-dimethylbenz(a)-anthracene in Sprague Dawley rats. Br J Cancer 1973 (27):63-71
34 Robinson SP, Jordan VC: Reversal of the antitumour effects of tamoxifen by progesterone in the 7,12-dimethylbenzanthracene-induced rat mammary carcinoma model. Cancer Res 1987 (47):5386-5390
35 Robinson SP, Mauel DA, Jordan VC: Antitumour actions of toremifene in the 7,12-dimethylbenzanthracene (DMBA)-induced rat

mammary tumor model. Eur J Cancer Clin Oncol 1988 (24):1817-1821
36 Gottardis MM, Jordan VC: Development of tamoxifen-stimulated growth of MCF-7 tumors in athymic mice after long-term antiestrogen administration. Cancer Res 1988 (48):5183-5187
37 Osborne CK, Coronado EB, Robinson JP: Human breast cancer in the athymic nude mouse: cytostatic effects of long-term antioestrogen therapy. Eur J Cancer Clin Oncol 1987 (23):1189-1196
38 Gottardis MM, Wagner RJ, Bordon EC, Jordan VC: Differential ability of antiestrogens to stimulate breast cancer cell (MCF-7) growth in vivo and in vitro. Cancer Res 1989 (49):4765-4769
39 Gottardis MM, Jiang SY, Jeng MH, Jordan VC: Inhibition of tamoxifen-stimulated growth of an MCF-7 tumor variant in athymic mice by novel steroidal antiestrogens. Cancer Res 1989 (49):4090-4093
40 Murray RML, Pitt P: Aminoglutethimide in tamoxifen-resistant patients: the Melbourne experience. Cancer Res 1982 (42 Suppl):3437s-3441s
41 Wakeling AE, Bowler J: Steroidal pure antioestrogens. J Endocrinol 1987 (112):R7-R10

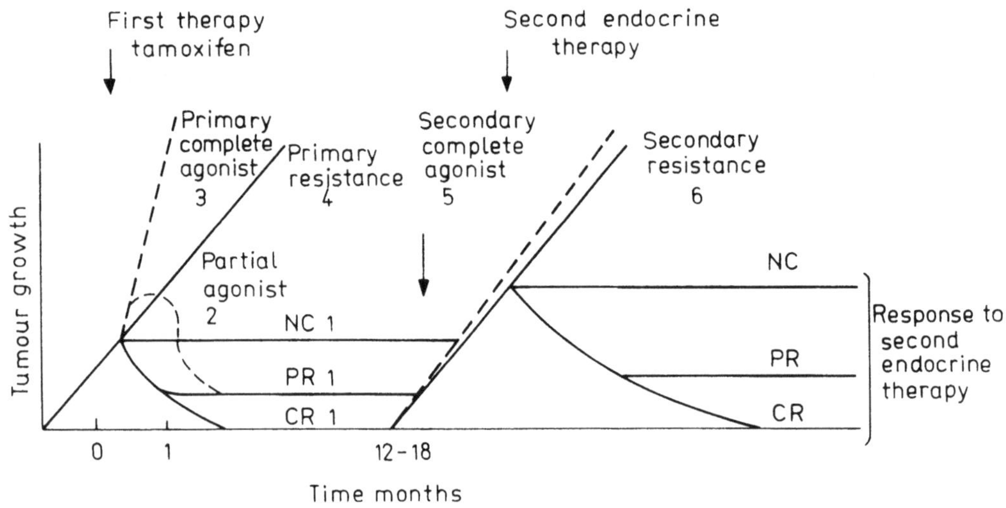


**Fig. 1.** Representation of the postulated possible types of response to tamoxifen in relation to duration of therapy and tumour growth. Tamoxifen when given as first therapy may cause: **1.** Regression (either NC {no change}, PR {partial remission} or CR {complete remission}). **2.** It may act as a partial agonist initially and produce a flare response before remission occurs. **3.** It may act as a complete agonist and continue to stimulate growth. **4.** The tumour may be primarily resistant. At regrowth after a remission on tamoxifen, we suggest that the drug may change from a complete antagonist (remission inducing) to a complete agonist to stimulate regrowth (**5**). The tumour may also regrow because of complete resistance to tamoxifen or any other endocrine therapy (**6**)

suggest that there are two possible further scenarios:

5. Tamoxifen changes from being a complete antagonist to being a complete agonist and *stimulates* tumour regrowth.
6. Tumour cells become completely resistant to tamoxifen and all other endocrine therapies: secondary complete resistance.

## Clinical and Experimental Data to Support the Six Types of Effect

### *Complete Antagonist*

The response rates to all first-line endocrine therapies are similar and are usually quoted as one-third of an unselected population of patients [13]. However, clinical data indicate that the response rate is nearer 50% because of the importance of the "no change" category of response as described in the UICC criteria by Hayward et al. [14]. When human mammary tumour cell lines (e.g., MCF-7) are induced to grow to form tumours by stimulation with oestrogen in nude mice, they respond to tamoxifen by stabilisation of growth only: partial or complete remissions are not seen in this model system [15,16]. Similarly, there is a group of patients where previously growing tumours are growth inhibited but they remain unchanged in size during treatment. The duration of tumour stabilisation which qualifies for a "no change" (NC) response differs between investigators. If a very short duration is taken, it may be difficult to distinguish between slow progression and NC because of the errors of measurement. We have suggested that the period should be 6 months. To a large extent this is arbitrary, but we have shown that, if this period is taken, the durations of NC and survival from the start of treatment are similar to patients who have a PR (Table 1, Fig. 2) [17]. Further evidence for the appropriateness of the NC category is the similarity in the proportions of receptor-positive tumours between NC and PR and the marked difference in proportion from those in patients who have progressive disease (Table 1). If we take NC as defined above as a "response" to therapy, then the overall response rate to tamoxifen is greater than 50% since over 20% of patients fall into the NC category .

**Table 1.** Data to indicate the similarity in response rate, median time to progression, median survival and oestrogen and progesterone receptor status in patients with partial responses and those in the "no change" category. All patients (n=267) had advanced disease and were treated with tamoxifen as first endocrine therapy. None were previously treated with any systemic therapy

| Response | Complete | Partial | No change | Progression |
|---|---|---|---|---|
| Number of patients (%) | 22 (8) | 65 (24) | 60 (22) | 120 (45) |
| Median time to progression (m) | 27 | 17 | 20 | 3 |
| Median survival (m) | 80 | 44 | 41 | 16 |
| ER +ve (%) | 16/19* (84) | 29/35 (83) | 32/38 (84) | 47/88 (53) |
| PR +ve (%) | 14/19 (74) | 23/35 (66) | 27/39 (69) | 27/88 (31) |

* receptors were not measured in all patients

## *Partial Agonist at Low Concentrations*

A small proportion of patients have an exacerbation of symptoms known as a flare response soon after treatment is started [7]. Three manifestations of the flare response have been described; increased growth, erythema or itching in soft tissue lesions, increased bone pain or hypercalcaemia. Since it takes more than 14 days, after initiation of oral therapy with tamoxifen, for steady-state serum levels to be reached, it is assumed that tamoxifen and its metabolites at relatively low concentrations are agonists for some tumours and become antagonists at pharmacological concentrations. An indication that the flare response is a true effect and not simply rapid tumour progression, is its close temporal association with the start of therapy with tamoxifen. Another indication of validity is the abrogation of the flare response by prednisolone. In a phase III trial comparing tamoxifen and tamoxifen with prednisolone as first systemic treatment for advanced breast cancer, Stewart et al. [18] reported 8 flare responses of 72 patients treated with tamoxifen alone, whereas there were none in the 73 patients treated with tamoxifen and prednisolone. Thus, it is probable that the partial agonist effect of tamoxifen is sufficient to produce symptoms in up to 10% of patients [13]. It may be a partial agonist for growth in most responding tumours but we have no methods for detecting this effect if symptoms are absent. However, we have previously demonstrated that tamoxifen is a partial agonist with respect to stimulaton of progesterone receptor (PR) synthesis in most patients who go on to respond to therapy [19].

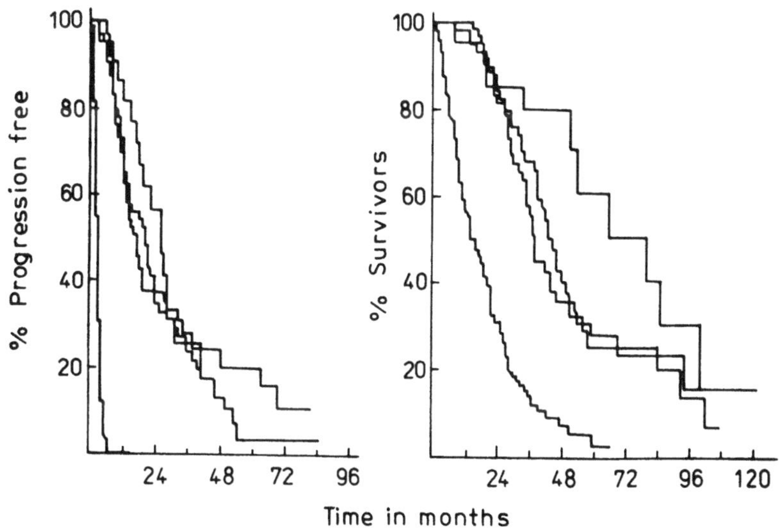


**Fig. 2.** Time to progression (left) and survival (right) from the time of start of tamoxifen therapy in 267 patients with advanced breast cancer. None had any previous systemic therapy. The 4 lines represent progressive disease (left-hand curve n = 120), no change (n = 60) and partial remission (n = 65: the virtually superimposable middle two curves), and complete remissions (n = 22: right-hand curve)

Several investigatiors have demonstrated an agonist effect of tamoxifen or its metabolites on the growth of oestrogen-responsive mammary tumour cell lines *in vitro*. The growth of the ZR-75-1 line was growth stimulated at a tamoxifen concentration of $10^{-7}$M [20]. In the ZR-75 line of Reddel and Sutherland [21], growth was stimulated at $10^{-9}$M. MCF-7 cells increased proliferation in the presence of $10^{-7}$M tamoxifen [22] and at $10^{-10}$M growth was stimulated by 4 hydroxy-tamoxifen, a major metabolite of tamoxifen [23]. At higher drug concentrations $\geq 10^{-6}$M, growth was inhibited in all the above reports.

The concentrations of tamoxifen and its metabolites in serum were reported by Etienne et al. [24]. At one hour after an oral dose, the serum concentration of tamoxifen was $1.7 \pm 0.5 \times 10^{-7}$M and at steady state it was $4.7 \pm 10^{-7}$M. The concentration of the metabolite, N desmethyl tamoxifen, at one hour was $0.04 \pm 0.01 \times 10^{-6}$M and $1.0 \pm 0.6 \times 10^{-6}$M after 8 weeks. These data indicate that, early in therapy, tamoxifen and its metabolites are at serum concentrations which *in vitro*, in some systems, may stimulate mammary tumour cell growth: late in therapy, serum levels of tamoxifen and its metabolites reach concentrations that would be inhibitory to cell growth.

Additional evidence for the partial agonist activity of tamoxifen and its metabolites is their effect on oestrogen-induced gene expression. These include expression of progesterone receptor, cathepsin D, plasminogen activator and a number of RNAs including pS2, pNR-100, pNR-1 and pNR-25 (see [25] for details). Tamoxifen at certain concentrations has similar effects as oestrogen on the expression of these proteins or RNAs. Interestingly, 4 metabolites of tamoxifen were also agonistic for all or some of the oestrogen-induced proteins or RNAs in the study reported by Johnson et al. [25].

### Complete Agonist De Novo

The evidence that tamoxifen can be a complete agonist when patients are first treated with the drug is indirect and principally derives from clinical observations. These are: (a) measurement of increase of tumour size; (b) flare responses which, when the drug is continued, do not result in tumour regression; (c) withdrawal responses to tamoxifen seen after the drug has been given for a short period only; (d) responses to second endocrine therapy after no response to tamoxifen, and (e) in addition there is evidence that tamoxifen is an agonist at sites other than the tumour, such as bone [26-28], the liver [29], and the genital tract [30,31].

#### *Increase in Tumour Size*

There is little objective evidence in the clinical literature that tamoxifen stimulates tumour growth. This, in part, may be due to the difficulty of collecting data which are unequivocal. Data on the growth rate before starting tamoxifen, during treatment and after cessation of treatment, are required to be reasonably certain of a growth effect of the drug. The patient reported by Legault-Poisson et al. [6] is most convincing in this regard. This patient had had no previous endocrine therapy. During spontaneous growth, the doubling time of her lung metastasis, as judged by serial chest x-rays, was 120 days. After starting tamoxifen, the doubling time decreased to 52 days. Treatment was discontinued after 110 days of therapy. One month later, progression of the tumour was still evident. The patient was kept off all anti-tumour therapy and there was then a gradual decline in tumour size to a partial remission. This remission lasted for 6+ months. These results suggest that the growth of the tumour was stimulated by tamoxifen *de novo* and also that the patient had a withdrawal response (WR) after cessation of therapy.

#### *Flare Response with No Tumour Regression after Continued Treatment with Tamoxifen*

It is stated that a flare response is an indication that patients will respond to subsequent continuation of the drug, provided the induced symptoms can be controlled for a period [32]. However, this is not always true. For example, in the trial comparing diethylstilboestrol (DES) with tamoxifen reported by Ingle et al. [2], 3 of 74 patients in the DES arm had a flare reaction and one responded when DES was continued. Two of 69 patients in the tamoxifen arm had a flare and one responded to continued treatment. None of the 8 patients reported to have a flare response to tamoxifen by Stewart et al. [18] went on to respond to tamoxifen. It is possible, but by no means proven, that failure to respond to continued tamoxifen after a flare response indicates that tamoxifen is acting as a complete agonist. It would be of interest to know the response to withdrawal of tamoxifen in this situation since we would predict which patients would respond.

### *Withdrawal Responses*

Withdrawal responses or "rebound regressions" have been reported after cessation of therapy with androgens [33], oestrogens [34] and tamoxifen [6]: the case described above was the first report of the WR to tamoxifen). Since 1979, several other reports of WR to tamoxifen have appeared [8-12]. Kaufman and Escher [35] were the first to report WRs in patients who had *not* responded to initial endocrine therapy (androgen or oestrogen). For tamoxifen, the case of Legault-Poisson et al. [6] was the first and we have seen 5 WR (30%) in 15 patients who had not had a response to tamoxifen. It is possible that, in all these cases where there was no response to initial endocrine therapy but a response when treatment was stopped, the tumour was stimulated *de novo* by tamoxifen acting as a complete agonist.

### *Response to Second Endocrine Therapy after No Response to Tamoxifen*

One of the unexplained paradoxes of endocrine therapy are responses to second therapy. Table 2 shows data on a group of 89 patients who were treated with tamoxifen and later with aromatase inhibitors or progestogens and who were evaluable for response to both treatments. Twenty-three of 55 (42%) patients who responded to first treatment with tamoxifen responded to second therapy. These data are most surprising when second responses to aminoglutethimide after tamoxifen are considered, since both drugs appear to act by reducing the amount of oestrogen "seen" by the tumour cell. Perhaps even more paradoxical are responses to second therapy even after there has been no response to the first. In this series, 5 of 34 (15%) patients who did not respond to first therapy responded to the second. This phenomenon has been well documented by others [13]. As with the WRs seen after no response to therapy with tamoxifen, it is possible that tamoxifen is acting as an agonist *de novo* and second therapy is antagonising its oestrogenic effect.

### *Other Agonist Effects of Tamoxifen*

It is of interest that tamoxifen acts as a pure agonist in the mouse. There is strong evidence that it acts as an agonist in sites other than mammary tumours in women with breast cancer. This is shown by the rise in SHBG [29], oestrogenic effects on serum lipids [36], prevention of osteoporosis [26-28], cornification of vaginal smears [31], the production of uterine fibroids [30], and stimulation of the endometrium [37,38] by tamoxifen treatment. It is perhaps not surprising, in the light of such evidence for extensive agonist activity in normal tissues, that there may well be primary agonist effects against some metastatic mammary tumours.

## Complete Resistance to Tamoxifen

Anaplastic, receptor-negative tumours are usually unresponsive to tamoxifen or any other type of endocrine therapy. Additional reasons for *de-novo* resistance to endocrine therapy may include the origin of some tumours from myoepithelial-like cells which do

**Table 2.** Response to second endocrine therapy (mainly aromatase inhibitors and progestogens) after treatment with tamoxifen as first therapy in 89 patients evaluable for both treatments

| | | RESPONSE TO SECOND 28/89 = 31% | | | |
|---|---|---|---|---|---|
| | | CR | PR | NC | PD |
| RESPONSE | CR | 1 | 2 | 0 | 3 |
| TO FIRST | PR | 0 | 2 | 4 | 15 |
| 55/89 = 62% | NC | 0 | 7 | 7 | 14 |
| | PD | 0 | 5 | 0 | 29 |

not contain receptors, loss of receptors or endocrine response elements of DNA or autonomous production of autocrine growth factors. From the discussions outlined above, *de-novo* resistance to endocrine therapy may occur only in about 40% of patients. Approximately 50% respond to tamoxifen (CR+PR+NC) and 10-15% of the total number of patients respond to second endocrine therapy when there is no response (or an agonist effect) to first-line treatment with tamoxifen.

### *Mechanisms of Regrowth after Response to Tamoxifen: Change to Complete Agonist?*

In the series of 267 patients reported in Table 1 treated with tamoxifen, the overall response rate was 54%, with a median duration of response of 20 months. After remission, the tumours of all responders regrew. However, 42% of tumours that originally responded to tamoxifen, responded to second endocrine therapy (Table 2). In order to account for second responses, we suggest that, after acting as an antagonist for a period of time, tamoxifen becomes an agonist. If this were the case, we would expect there to be withdrawal responses to tamoxifen in this situation as well as the well-documented responses to second endocrine therapy.

Recently, we (Dodwell et al. [10]) reviewed a group of 53 patients who had responded to tamoxifen and at progression the only "therapy" given was to withdraw tamoxifen. Twelve patients had either a partial remission or "no change" for an overall response rate of 23% (Table 3). The median duration of remission for WR was 11 months, which is equivalent in length of time to the duration of additive second endocrine therapies in our experience. The patients whom we assessed for WR tended to have slow growing soft-tissue disease and, as such, represented a selected population. However, the data indicate that PRs or prolonged stabilisation of disease can occur after initial response to tamoxifen followed by simply stopping the drug and suggest that tamoxifen had become an agonist after it had been shown to be an antagonist.

Animal data to support the change of tamoxifen from antagonist to agonist during prolonged remissons are demonstrated in the experiments reported by Gottardis et al. [15,16]. The growth of MCF-7 cells in nude mice was inhibited for several months by tamoxifen. However, after this period, the tumour growth rate increased in spite of continued therapy with tamoxifen. After withdrawal of tamoxifen from the animals, growth of the tumour stopped, which suggests that tamoxifen had become an agonist. In this model, oestrogen receptors increased and were certainly not lost during the transition from growth inhibition to growth stimulation by tamoxifen. However, when the tamoxifen-stimulated cells were removed from the mice and grown *in vitro*, they could then be inhibited by tamoxifen. Thus, the growth stimulation *in vivo* by tamoxifen in the mice may be by an indirect mechanism.

A second experiment which supports the notion that tamoxifen may change from an antagonist to an agonist *in vivo* was reported by Simon et al. [39]. They took tumour cells from pleural effusions from 2 patients who had responded to tamoxifen but then progressed. The tumour cells were grown in serum-free medium in the presence of $10^{-6}$M tamoxifen and under these conditions growth of each line was stimulated by 40-45% over a 5-day culture period. Both lines were stimulated by

**Table 3.** Withdrawal responses after cessation of therapy with tamoxifen

| | No. | No. with WR | (%) |
|---|---|---|---|
| Initial response to tamoxifen | 42 | 14 | 33 |
| No initial response to tamoxifen | 15 | 5 | 30 |
| Treated with tamoxifen but not evaluable for response | 14 | 4 | 29 |

**Table 4.** Details of 2 patients with repeated responses to tamoxifen and a withdrawal response. Both patients had relatively indolent chest wall recurrences with no evident disease at other sites during endocrine therapy

| | Mrs A | Mrs B |
|---|---|---|
| Age: | 54 | 72 |
| | Durations and type of response (months) | |
| Tamoxifen | 57 (CR) | 27 (CR) |
| Withdrawal | 11 (NC) | 20 (NC) |
| Tamoxifen | 7 (PR) | 6 (PR) |
| Withdrawal | - (PD) | - (PD) |
| Course | Liver metastases given chemotherapy | No response to 4OH androstenedione |

$10^{-8}$ M oestradiol to the same extent as by $10^{-6}$ M tamoxifen. Both patients were withdrawn from tamoxifen treatment and both had a WR. The stimulation of tumour cells *in vitro* suggests that this may have occurred *in vivo* and accounted for disease progression. This suggestion is supported by the clinical WRs seen after stopping tamoxifen.

The change of how tumour cells "see" tamoxifen may alter more than once. This is suggested by 2 patients we have studied. Their clinical course suggests that a switch from agonist to antagonist may be reversible (Table 4). Both patients developed soft-tissue recurrences on the chest wall and had prolonged complete remissions (57 and 27 months, respectively) to tamoxifen, which was given continuously. When the disease progressed, tamoxifen was withdrawn. Both patients then had a WR with disease NC for 11 and 20, months respectively. On progression, there were further partial remissions (7 and 6 months, respectively) after the reintroduction of tamoxifen. The patients then failed to respond to a second withdrawal of tamoxifen and had no further endocrine responses. The site of progression after initial complete response to tamoxifen was of the original chest wall disease. A WR suggests that tamoxifen may have become an agonist. However, after a prolonged period of WR it appeared that tamoxifen was able to act as an antagonist again.

Change from an antagonist to agonist may be only one mechanism of "resistance" to tamoxifen. Van den Berg et al. [40] grew ZR-75-1 cells in progressively increasing concentrations of tamoxifen until the cells became resistant and grew well in the presence of tamoxifen. At this time, oestrogen and progesterone receptors were no longer detectable. The cells were then grown in the absence of tamoxifen. After 4 weeks, the cells acquired ER and PR again and regained their sensitivity to the antagonist effects of tamoxifen. It does not appear from these experiments that tamoxifen became an agonist.

## *Secondary Complete Resistance*

After initial response to tamoxifen followed by regrowth, approximately 50% of patients have no WR or response to any other endocrine therapy. The mechanism of this secondary resistance is not clear. Long-term growth of MCF-7 cells in the presence of tamoxifen results in the emergence of cell lines apparently completely resistant to tamoxifen [41-43]. However, in these experiments oestrogen and progesterone receptors were not lost and the cells still responded to oestrogen by an increase in progesterone receptor synthesis but did not respond with respect to growth. This suggests that the receptor-ligand complex interacts at a different point on the genome for growth and for non growth-related events. But the effect of tamoxifen on proliferation after "resistance" had been acquired was not tested; it is possible that tamoxifen had become an agonist in this model. It is, therefore, not known whether the secondary complete resistance that is clearly seen *in vivo* is demonstrable *in vitro*. This comment does not apply to the receptor-negative cell lines which are clearly resistant to pharmacological concentrations of tamoxifen. Although there is a trend towards loss of receptors with time, *in vivo* several groups have shown that resistance to tamoxifen was not always associated with receptor loss [44-46].

## Conclusions

In this chapter we have summarised the possible types of response and lack of response to tamoxifen which can occur in patients with advanced breast cancer.

Although some of the differences in response could be explained by differences in metabolism of the tamoxifen between patients or with time in individual patients, there are no data to support this hypothesis. The recent paper by Etienne et al. [24] shows that there are no significant differences in serum levels of tamoxifen, or any of the metabolites measured, between patients who responded and non-responders.

There is evidence that there are marked differences in the way that cells see tamoxifen between species and between tissues in a single species. The data summarised above also indicate that whether tamoxifen acts as an agonist or an antagonist can depend on the drug concentration and the duration of exposure of the tissues. The agonist effect at low concentrations may explain the so-called tumour "flare" response seen at the start of treatment in some patients. The data summarised above also suggest that tamoxifen may be a complete agonist *de novo* in tumours or change from antagonist to agonist after a prolonged period of treatment. It is not clear whether this change occurs within the tumour cell (as the Simon experiments suggest) or as a change in the way other non-tumour cells see tamoxifen, which then secondarily alters tumour-cell proliferation (as the Gottardis nude mouse experiments suggest).

What implications do the observations and hypotheses outlined above have for patient management? Endocrine therapy for advanced disease is palliative, but any measures we can take to improve response rate and prolong response for as long as possible would be of value. The arguments put forward here have several implications for improved therapy.

1. Treatment should not be changed until there is definite evidence of progression of disease since NC is a response.
2. In the absence of life-threatening disease, it can be worth looking for a WR to tamoxifen if there has been no initial response, or at relapse after previous response. Remissions last on average as long as responses to second endocrine therapy, especially if there is soft tissue disease only.
3. The duration of response to tamoxifen could be extended by measures which prevent a change to agonism or resistance. Darbre and King [47] have demonstrated that progression to insensitivity to androgens *in vitro* can be prevented by culture in the presence of corticosteroids. The presence of prednisolone also appears to extend the period of responsiveness and survival with tamoxifen treatment compared with tamoxifen alone in women with advanced breast cancer [48]. Resistance may also be reduced by treatment with tamoxifen intermittently: a hypothesis which is currently being tested by the EORTC.
4. The appropriate test of the hypothesis that the agonist activity of antioestrogens may lower their effectiveness as anti-tumour agents is to compare them in the clinic with anti-oestrogens which do not have agonist activity [23]. We predict that such agents would be associated with higher response rates and longer response durations compared with partial agonist anti-oestrogens.

## REFERENCES

1 Cole MP, Jones CTA andTodd IDH: A new anti-oestrogenic agent in late breast cancer: an early clinical appraisal of ICI 46474. Br J Cancer 1971 (25):270-275

2 Ingle JN, Ahmann DL, Green SJ et al: Randomized clinical trial of diethylstilboestrol versus tamoxifen in postmenopausal women with advanced breast cancer: N Engl J Med 1981 (304):16-21

3 Buchanan RB, Blamey RW, Durrant KR et al: A randomized comparison of tamoxifen with surgical oophorectomy in premenopausal patients with advanced breast cancer. J Clin Oncol 1986 (49):1326-1330

4 Early Breast Trialist's Collaborative Group: Effect of adjuvant tamoxifen and of cytotoxic therapy on mortality in early breast cancer. N Engl J Med 1988 (319):1681-1692

5 Report from Scottish Breast Cancer Trials: Adjuvant tamoxifen in the management of operable breast cancer. The Scottish Trial. Lancet 1987 (ii):171-175

6 Legault-Poisson S, Jolivet J, Poisson R et al: Tamoxifen-induced tumor stimulation and withdrawal response. Cancer Treat Rep 1979 (63):1839-1841

7 Clarysse A: Hormone-induced tumor flare: Eur J Cancer Clin Oncol 1985 (21):545-547

8 Rudolph R: Response of metastatic breast cancer to tamoxifen (TAM) withdrawal: Proc Am Soc Oncol 1986 (5):270

9 Canney PA, Griffiths T, Latief TN et al: Clinical significance of tamoxifen withdrawal response. Lancet 1987 (i):36

10 Dodwell DJ, Howell A and Anderson H: Withdrawal responses to tamoxifen. Submitted for publication

11 Belani CP, Pearl P, Whitley NO: Tamoxifen withdrawal response. Arch Intern Med 1989 (149):449-450

12 Stein W, Hortobagyl GN and Blumanschein GR: Response of metastatic breast cancer to tamoxifen withdrawal: a report of a case. J Surg Oncol 1983 (22):45-46

13 Henderson I Craig: Endocrine therapy in metastatic breast cancer. In: Harris JR, Hellman S, Henderson IC, Kinne DW (eds) Breast Diseases. JB Lippincott Co, Philadelphia 1987 p 398

14 Hayward JI, Carbone PP, Heuson JC et al : Assessment of response to therapy in advanced breast cancer . Eur J Cancer 1977 (13):89-94

15 Gottardis MM, Jiang SY, Jeng MH and Craig Jordon V: Inhibition of tamoxifen-stimulated growth of an MCF-7 tumour variant in athymic mice by novel steroidal antiestrogens. Cancer Res 1989 (49):4090-4093

16 Gottardis MM, Wagner RJ, Borden EC and Craig Jordon V: Differential ability of antiestrogens to stimulate breast cancer cell (MCF-7) growth in vivo and in vitro. Cancer Res 1989 (49):4765-4769

17 Howell A, Harland RNL, Barnes DM, Hayward E, Redford J: Endocrine therapy for advanced carcinoma of the breast: the relationship between the effect of tamoxifen upon concentrations of progesterone receptor and subsequent response to treatment: Cancer Res 1987 (47):300-304

18 Stewart JF, Rubens RD, King RJB et al: Contribution of prednisolone to the primary endocrine treatment of advanced breast cancer: Eur J Cancer Clin Oncol 1982 (18):1307-1314

19 Howell A, Harland RNL, Barnes DM et al: Endocrine therapy for advanced carcinoma of the breast: the effect of tumour heterogeneity and site of biopsy upon the predictive value of progesterone receptor estimations. Cancer Res 1987 (47):296-299

20 Darbre PD, Curtis S,and King RJB: Effects of oestradiol and tamoxifen on human breast cancer cells in serum-free culture: Cancer Res 1984(44):2790-2793

21 Reddel RR and Sutherland RL: Tamoxifen stimulation of human breast cancer cell proliferation in vitro: a possible model for tamoxifen tumour flare. Eur J Cancer Clin Oncol 1984 (11):1419-1424

22 Roos W, Huber P, Oeze L and Eppenberger U: Hormone dependency and the action of tamoxifen in human mammary carcinoma cells. Anticancer Res 1982 (2):157-162

23 Wakeling AE, Newboult E and Peters SW: Effects of antioestrogens on the proliferation of MCF-7 human breast cancer cells. J Mol Endocrinol 1989 (2):1-10

24 Etienne MC, Milano G, Fischel JL et al: Tamoxifen metabolism: pharmokinetic and in-vitro study. Br J Cancer 1989 (60):30-35

25 Johnson MD, Westley BR, and May FEB : Oestrogenic activity of tamoxifen and its metabolites on gene regulation and cell proliferation in MCF-7 breast cancer cells. Br J Cancer 1989 (59):727-738

26 Love RR, Mazess RB, Tormey DC et al: Bone mineral density (BMD) in women with breast cancer treated with tamoxifen for two years. Breast Cancer Res Treat 1988 (12):297-302

27 Fentiman IS, Caleffi M, Murby B and Fogelman I: Dosage, duration and short term effect on bone mineral content of tamoxifen treatment for mastalgia. Br J Clin Pract 1988 (52 S56):18

28 Turken S, Siris E, Seldin D et al: Effects of tamoxifen on spinal bone density in women with breast cancer: JNCI 1989 (81):1086-1088

29 Jordan VC, Fritz NF and Tormey DC: Long-term adjuvant therapy with tamoxifen effects on sex hormone binding globulin and anti-thrombin III. Cancer Res 1987 (47):4517-4519

30 Boudouris O, Ferrand S, Guillet JL and Madelenat P: Effets pardoxaux du tamoxifene sur l'utérus de la femme. J Gynecol Obstet Biol Reprod 1989 (18):372-378

31 Boccardo F, Bruzzi P, Rubagotti A et al: Oestrogen like action of tamoxifen on vaginal epithelium in breast cancer patients. Rev Endo Rel Cancer 1981 (S9):242-250

32 Villalon A, Tattersall M, Fox R and Woods R: Hypercalcaemia after tamoxifen for breast cancer: a sign of tumour response. Br Med J 1979 (2):1329-1330

33 Escher GC: Clinical improvement of inoperable breast carcinoma under steroid treatment. Proc 1st Conference on Steroid Hormones and Mammary Carcinoma, April 1949 pp 92-99

34 Huesby RA: Estrogen therapy in the management of advanced breast carcinoma. Am J Surg 1954

(20):112-115
35 Kaufman RJ and Escher GC: Rebound regression in advanced mammary carcinoma. Surg Gynecol Obstet 1961 (113):635-640
36 Powles TJ, Hardy JR, Ashley SE et al: A pilot trial to evaluate the acute toxicity and feasibility of tamoxifen for prevention of breast cancer: Br J Cancer 1989 (60):126-131
37 Jordan VC: Tamoxifen and endometrial cancer: Lancet 1988 (ii):1019
38 Gottardis MM, Robinson SP, Satayaswaroop PG and Craig Jordan V: Contrasting actions of tamoxifen on endometrial and breast tumour growth in the athymic mouse. Cancer Res 1988 (48):812-814
39 Simon WE, Albrecht M, Trams G et al: In vitro growth promotion of human mammary carcinoma cells by steroid hormones, tamoxifen, and prolactin. JNCI 1984 (73):313-321
40 Van den Berg HW, Lynch M, Martin J et al: Characterisation of a tamoxifen-resistant variant of the ZR-75-1 human breast cancer cell line ( ZR-75-9a1) and stability of the resistant phenotype. Br J Cancer 1989 (59):522-526
41 Bronzert DA, Greene GL and Lippman ME: Selection and characterization of a breast cancer cell line resistant to the antiestrogen LY 117018. Endocrinology 1985 (117):1409-1417
42 Nawata H, Bronzert D and Lippman ME: Isolation and characterization of a tamoxifen-resistant cell line derived from MCF-7 human breast cancer cells. J Biol Chem 1981 (256):5016-5021
43 Nawata H, Chong MT, Bronzert D and Lippman ME: Estradiol-independent growth of MCF-7 human breast cancer cells in culture. J Biol Chem 1981 (256):6895-6902
44 Toma S, Leonessa F and Paridaens R: The effects of therapy on estrogen receptors in breast cancer. J Steroid Biochem 1985 (23):1105-1109
45 Crawford DJ, Cowan S, Fitch R et al: Stability of oestrogen receptor status in sequential biopsies from patients with breast cancer: Br J Cancer 1987 (56):137-140
46 Henry JA, Nicholson S, Hennessy C et al: Expression of the oestrogen regulated pNR-2mRNA in human breast cancer. Relation to oestrogen receptor mRNA levels and response to tamoxifen therapy. Br J Cancer 1990 (61):32-38
47 Darbre PD and King RJB: Progression to steroid insensitivity can occur irrespective of the presence of functional steroid receptors. Cell 1987 (51):521-528
48 Rubens RD, Tinson CL, Coleman RE et al: Prednisolone improves the response to primary endocrine treatment for advanced breast cancer: Br J Cancer 1988 (58):626-630

# A Review of the International Experience with the LHRH Agonist Zoladex in the Treatment of Advanced Breast Cancer in Pre- and Perimenopausal Women

R.A.V. Milsted and M.J. Matthews

Medical Research Department, ICI Pharmaceuticals, Alderley Park, Macclesfield, Cheshire, United Kingdom

Since the work of Beatson [1], the established basis for the palliative treatment of advanced breast cancer in pre- and perimenopausal women has been ovarian ablation, either by surgery or by irradiation.

"Zoladex" * (goserelin) is a luteinising hormone releasing hormone (LHRH) agonist which, on continuous administration, suppresses release of gonadotrophins by downregulation of the pituitary LHRH receptors [2]. Reduction in luteinising hormone (LH) production by the anterior pituitary gland brings about a consequent reduction in oestrogen production by the ovary, resulting in serum oestradiol levels comparable to those observed following ovarian ablation.

"Zoladex" has been investigated as a treatment for advanced breast cancer because it appeared to offer a medical alternative to ovarian ablation. The data reported here are believed to represent the largest single coordinated programme of study of the treatment of advanced breast cancer in pre- and perimenopausal women.

## Patients and Methods

### *Patients*

Between 21 July 1982 and 19 August 1988, 265 pre- and perimenopausal patients with advanced (metastatic) breast cancer were treated with "Zoladex" 3.6 mg depot in 16 clinical trials of efficacy and safety in the U.K. and Europe. Thirty-two percent (74 patients) had received previous systemic therapy for breast cancer; in the majority (60 patients), this was adjuvant cytotoxic or hormone therapy. Patients receiving concomitant therapy that could affect sex hormones were excluded from the analysis of efficacy. Two hundred and twenty-eight patients were eligible for this analysis.

Safety data were collected from a total of 333 pre- and perimenopausal patients with breast cancer, comprising the 265 entered in the trials of efficacy and safety plus 68 patients entered in trials not analysed for efficacy because of protocol violations (e.g., daily injection formulation of "Zoladex" used; only patients with primary disease admitted) or because fewer than 5 patients were recruited.

### *Treatment*

In all the studies of efficacy, "Zoladex" was given as the 3.6 mg depot ("Zoladex depot" ICI Pharmaceuticals) injected subcutaneously into the anterior abdominal wall once every 28 days by pre-filled applicator. A daily injection formulation of "Zoladex" was in use before the depot became available, and 27 patients received only the daily injection.

### *Clinical Trials*

The clinical trials were open, non-comparative studies in which patients were assessed at regular intervals by clinical examination, symptom enquiry and the appropriate investi-

* "Zoladex" is a trademark, the property of Imperial Chemical Industries PLC.

gations in order to measure subjective, objective and endocrinological response, and tolerance.

Data from patients recruited less than 3 months before their study was closed for analysis are excluded to provide for at least 3 months' follow-up information on all patients contributing efficacy data.

Subjective clinical response was assessed by questioning at follow-up visits about any limitations to daily activities, pain, and analgesic use that were attributable to breast cancer. Improvement in one or more of these with no worsening in any was considered a subjective response.

Assessment of objective clinical response was based on the currently accepted Union Internationale Contre le Cancer (UICC) criteria [3].

Endocrine response was measured by determination of serum concentrations of LH and oestradiol at follow-up visits. A serum oestradiol value of 40 pg/ml was chosen as a representative upper limit of the postmenopausal range for oestradiol in the laboratories at the study centres.

The effect of "Zoladex" 3.6 mg depot on menstruation was also recorded.

Tolerance of the drug was assessed by recording adverse events and assessing the study data for evidence of certain pharmacological effects (hot flushes, changes in libido, headaches, vaginal dryness and changes in mood).

### *Analysis*

The clinical trials providing efficacy data followed a standard design which facilitated pooling of the data. Pooled rates were calculated for overall subjective and objective response. In all cases, the best objective response achieved during treatment was used in the analysis. Absence of objective progression with insufficient evidence of partial objective regression was classified as no change. No change was not considered to represent an objective response.

Median times to subjective response and objective response, median duration of response in responders and overall median time to progression also provide an assessment of clinical efficacy.

Results of hormone measurements are presented as means with standard deviations.

## Results

### *Endocrine Response*

*Serum LH*

Following an initial transient rise, the mean serum LH is suppressed after the administration of a single 3.6 mg depot of "Zoladex" once every 28 days (Fig. 1).

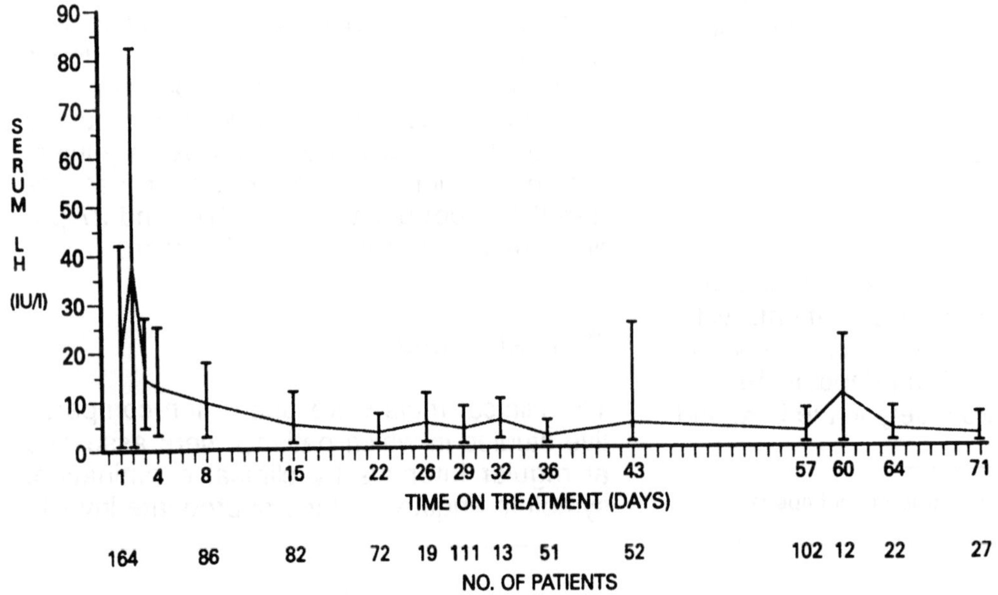


**Fig. 1.** Serum luteinising hormone concentration (mean and standard deviation) during the first 12 weeks of treatment

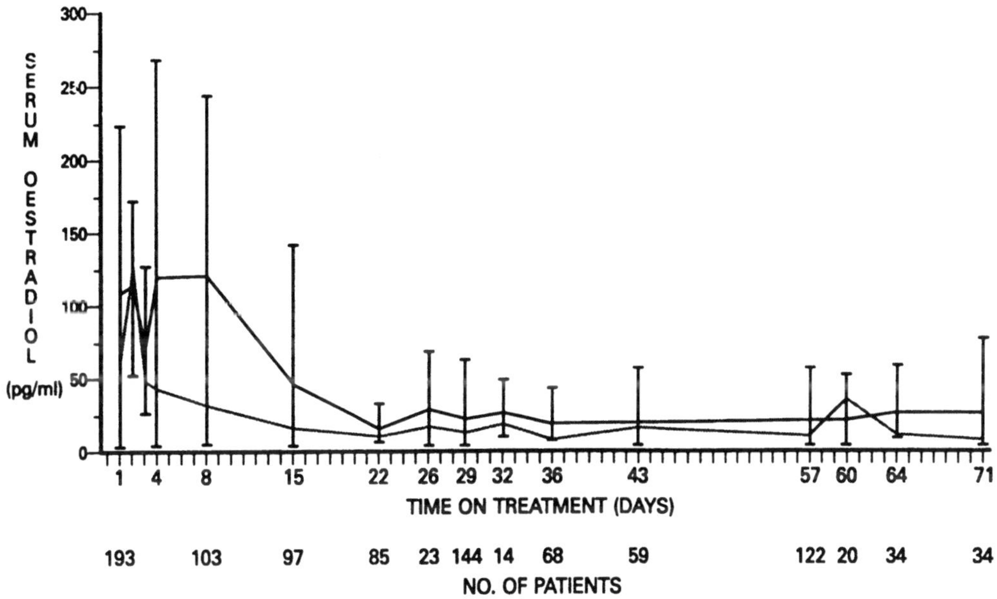


**Fig. 2.** Serum oestradiol concentration (mean and standard deviation) during the first 12 weeks of treatment

*Serum oestradiol*

The mean serum oestradiol concentration was suppressed to a value below 40 pg/ml by day 22 after the administration of a single 3.6 mg depot of "Zoladex" and remained suppressed thereafter (Fig. 2).

***Menstruation***

Menstruation occurred in 47% of assessed patients during the first 4 weeks of treatment. Table 1 shows the number and the percentage of patients who reported menstruation or an episode of PV bleeding subsequently.

In only 5 patients was menstruation or PV bleeding associated with a serum oestradiol concentration above 40 pg/ml after week 8.

***Subjective Clinical Response***

One hundred and forty-two patients were symptomatic at entry to the studies. Ninety-seven (68.3%) had a subjective response to "Zoladex" depot; the median time to subjective response was 8 weeks (range 1-52).

***Objective Clinical Response***

Eighty-three patients (36.4%) showed an objective clinical response (UICC Complete or Partial Response) to "Zoladex" depot. The median time to response among these patients was 12 weeks (range 4-49). The lifetable median duration of response was 44 weeks (range >4 - >160) (Fig. 3).

Objective clinical responses were observed in patients of all age groups studied, in all histological grades of tumour encountered, and regardless of oestrogen receptor (ER) status of the tumour (Table 2).

Objective clinical responses were observed in patients with either advanced disease at first diagnosis or recurrent disease at entry to the studies (assessed by disease-free interval, DFI) and in patients with previous adju-

**Table 1.** Menstruation/PV bleeding during treatment with "Zoladex"

| Weeks on treatment | Pts with PV bleed vs Pts assessed | Percentage with PV bleed |
|---|---|---|
| 8 | 12/197 | 6.1% |
| 12 | 10/168 | 5.9% |
| 16 | 1/52 | 1.9% |
| 20 | 1/41 | 2.4% |
| 24 | 3/91 | 3.3% |
| 28 | 1/31 | 3.2% |
| 36 | 2/62 | 3.2% |
| 60 | 1/25 | 4.0% |

PV = per vaginam

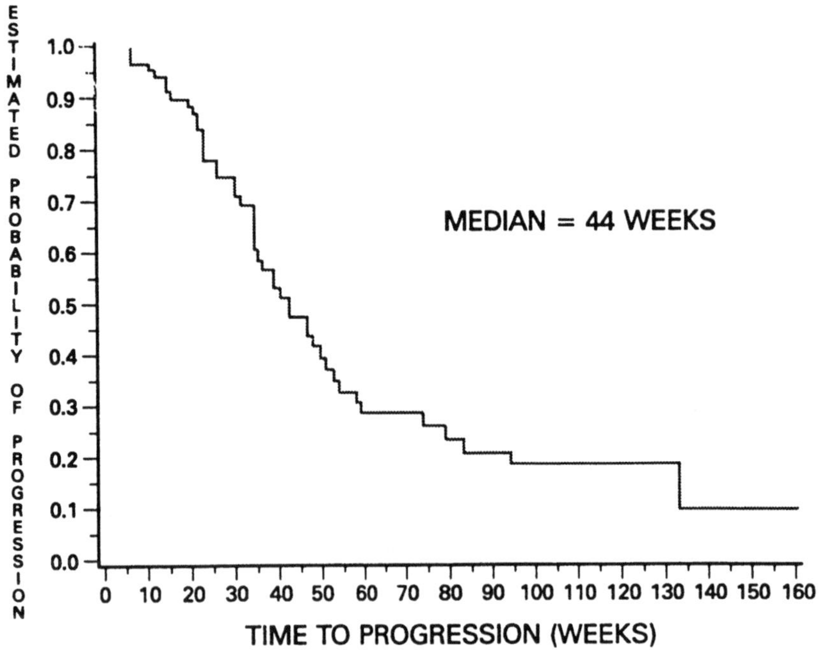


**Fig. 3.** Lifetable median duration of response in responding patients

vant therapy or hormone therapy for advanced disease (Table 3).

Thirty-two patients (14.0%) showed only disease progression during the studies. One hundred and sixty-three patients (71.5%) had had progression of disease at the time of the analysis. The lifetable median time to progression was 22 weeks (range 1 - >160) in all eligible patients.

## *Tolerability and Safety*

"Zoladex" depot was extremely well tolerated. Safety data were collected from 333 pre- and perimenopausal breast cancer patients. There were no suspected adverse reactions so severe as to require therapy to be withdrawn. The majority of the 58 possible adverse reactions reported in 34 patients were

**Table 2.** Objective clinical response rate to "Zoladex" by age of patient, histological grade and ER status

| Assessment | Classification | (n) | Objective Response (CR + PR) % |
|---|---|---|---|
| Overall | total assessed | (228) | 36.4 |
| Age (yrs) | below 36 | (37) | 32.4 |
| | 36-40 | (50) | 38.0 |
| | 41-45 | (77) | 37.7 |
| | over 45 | (64) | 35.9 |
| Tumour: degree of histological differentiation | | | |
| | high | (8) | 50.0 |
| | medium | (85) | 44.7 |
| | low | (69) | 26.1 |
| | unknown | (66) | 34.8 |
| ER status | positive | (102) | 44.1 |
| | negative | (49) | 30.6 |
| | unknown | (77) | 29.9 |

ER = oestrogen receptor; CR = complete response; PR = partial response

**Table 3.** Objective clinical response rate to "Zoladex" by previous history

| Factor | History | (n) | Objective response (CR + PR) % |
|---|---|---|---|
| DFI (months) | 0 | (38) | 36.8 |
| | 1-24 | (108) | 29.6 |
| | 25-48 | (54) | 48.1 |
| | over 48 | (28) | 39.3 |
| Previous hormone therapy for advanced disease | | | |
| | No | (214) | 37.4 |
| | Yes | (14) | 21.4 |
| Previous adjuvant therapy, no previous hormone therapy for advanced disease | | | |
| | No | (154) | 39.0 |
| | Yes | (60) | 33.3 |

CR = complete response; PR = partial response; DFI = disease-free interval

graded either mild or moderate in severity by the clinician. The most frequent possible adverse reactions were hot flushes and sweating (11 reports), nausea or nausea and vomiting (8) and dry mouth [5].

Local bruising or intolerance to the depot injection was rare (4 cases). Seven patients experienced a worsening of signs or symptoms during the first month of therapy. In 4 cases, this was associated with progression of breast cancer. In the other 3 cases, the symptoms resolved with analgesia, radiotherapy, or other specific management. Some of the pharmacological effects of oestrogen suppression were commonly encountered, but they were not often reported as possible adverse reactions (Table 4).

**Table 4.** Pharmacological effects of oestrogen suppression during treatment with "Zoladex"

| | Pts in whom recorded on treatment | Pts in whom reported as a possible adverse reaction |
|---|---|---|
| Onset of hot flushes | 154 | 10 |
| Decreased libido | 92 | 0 |
| Vaginal dryness | 2 | 1 |
| Headache | 6 | 5 |
| Mood change | 1 | 1 |

Of the 13 deaths reported, only 3 were attributable to causes other than breast cancer alone. These were: (i) pulmonary embolism after surgical decompression of spinal metastases, (ii) pneumonia in the presence of disseminated disease, (iii) acute pulmonary oedema with a history of heart disease requiring digoxin and frusemide.

## Discussion

The clinical response rate in pre- and perimenopausal women with advanced breast cancer following surgical ablation of the ovaries is in the range of 21%-37% [4-8]. The objective response rate (CR+PR) of 36.4% achieved with "Zoladex" depot as an initial treatment for advanced breast cancer in pre- and perimenopausal women compares very favourably with this, and with the response rates achieved in similar patient groups with the anti-oestrogen "Nolvadex" * (tamoxifen) (around 30%) with the same duration of response of around 12 months.

In premenopausal patients with advanced breast cancer, favourable prognostic factors for response to hormonal manipulation include ER-positive tumours, a long disease-

* "Nolvadex" is a trademark, the property of Imperial Chemical Industries PLC.

# Adjuvant Systemic Therapy in Node-Negative Breast Cancer

Manfred Kaufmann

Universitäts-Frauenklinik, Voss-Strasse 9, 6900 Heidelberg, F.R.G.

## Benefit from Adjuvant Systemic Therapy

After more than 40 years of experience with systemic adjuvant therapy and more than 100 reported randomised adjuvant trials in breast cancer, it can be stated that adjuvant treatment significantly changes the natural course of this systemic and chronic disease.

International overview data [1] of randomised trials (1967-1985) show prolongation of disease-free and overall survival at 5 years for adjuvant chemotherapy and adjuvant tamoxifen treatment, chiefly for node-positive tumours in pre- (<50 years) and postmenopausal (≥50 years) women (Table 1). Most benefit-risk analyses have been made for node-positive tumours and most effort has been focussed on this subset of breast cancers. Although the overview data on this subgroup of primary breast cancers are not only of statistical but also of medical significance, the most important objective, i.e., to cure operable breast cancer, has not been attained. During the past decade, the use of adjuvant treatment was, therefore, extended to include the subgroup of node-negative tumours.

Recommendations of a standard treatment for node-positive tumours were made in 1985 and revised in 1988 by Glick [2]. Outside of clinical trials, early guide-lines also applied to node-negative tumours. However, these suggestions are not based on analysed overview data and no clearly defined subgroups ("high-risk") have been established to date. The first randomised trials in node-negative operable breast cancer compared a surgical control and an adjuvant-treated group, as was the case in the initial trials with node-positive tumours.

**Table 1.** Effects of adjuvant cytotoxic (CMF ± other drugs) and endocrine (Tamoxifen) treatment on reduction of mortality

| | Survival at 5 years | |
|---|---|---|
| | < 50 years | ≥ 50 years |
| Surgery only | 66% | 66% |
| CMF ± drugs | 73% | 67% |
| - difference | 6.9% ± 2.0 | 1.2% ± 1.6 |
| Surgery only | 70% | 68% |
| Tamoxifen | 71% | 73% |
| - difference | 0.5% ± 1.9 | 5.9% ± 1.0 |

The early reported trials evaluating the efficiency of adjuvant chemotherapy (Table 2) or adjuvant tamoxifen (Table 3) mostly selected node-negative tumours for analysis, because both node-positive and node-negative tumours were included in these trials. This generally resulted in small numbers of patients, especially in the chemotherapy trials. Disease-free survival was improved for patients who received chemotherapy or tamoxifen. Survival benefits were not always apparent or were only transient, and probably smaller than those observed in node-positive tumours.

Four recently published trials included only patients with node-negative tumours and were accordingly larger. They also included prospectively defined risk subgroups. Their data resulted in a "Clinical Alert" published in the U.S.A. by the National Cancer Institute, and led to widespread and controversial discussion [3,4]. Two studies analysed 6-12 months of adjuvant chemotherapy [5,6]: one of them investigated a single course of peri-

**Table 2.** Published randomised trials of adjuvant chemotherapy in node-negative breast cancer before 1989

| Study | No. patients | Designs | DFS % | Follow-up (years) |
|---|---|---|---|---|
| Nissen-Meyer et al. [25] | 609 | control vs C* | 55<br>65 | 20 |
| Senn et al. [26] | 123 | control vs LMF+BCG x 6 | 62<br>68 | 10 |
| Morrison et al. [27] | 543 | control vs LMF x 8 | 74<br>75 | 5 |
| Jakesz et al. [28] | 128 | control vs CMF Vp ± Immune stim. | 77<br>84 | 6 |
| Bonadonna [3] | 90** | control vs CMF x 12 | 45<br>87 | 6 |

* perioperative; ** ER-negative tumours

**Table 3.** Published randomised trials of adjuvant tamoxifen in node-negative breast cancer before 1989

| Study | No. patients | Designs | DFS % | Follow-up (years) |
|---|---|---|---|---|
| Scottish Trial [29] | 751* | control vs Tam 20 mg 5 years | benefit n.s. | 8 |
| NATO [30] | 605 | control vs Tam 20 mg 5 years | benefit n.s. | 8 |
| CRC Trial [31] | 887 | control vs Tam 20 mg 2 years | benefit | 5 |
| Stockholm Trial [32] | 1323* | control vs Tam 40 mg 2-5 years | NA | 10 |

* postmenopausal; NA = not available; n.s. = not statistically significant; Tam = tamoxifen

**Table 4.** Recently published larger randomised trials of adjuvant chemotherapy or tamoxifen in node-negative breast cancer

| Study | No. patients | Designs | DFS % | Survival % | Follow-up (years) |
|---|---|---|---|---|---|
| NSABP B-13 [5] | 741* | control<br>vs<br>MF (leucov.) x 12 | 71<br>p=0.003<br>80 | 86<br>p=0.8<br>87 | 4 |
| Intergroup Trial [6] | 422 | control<br>vs<br>CMFP x 6 | 67<br>p=0.0001<br>84 | 88<br>p=0.3<br>91 | 3 |
| Ludwig Trial V [7] | 1275 | control<br>vs<br>CMF (leucov.) x 1 | 73<br>p=0.04<br>77 | 86<br>p=0.24<br>90 | 3.5 |
| NSABP B-14 [8] | 2644** | control<br>vs<br>Tam (5 years) | 77<br>p< 0.00001<br>83 | 92<br>p=0.3<br>93 | 4 |

* ER-negative tumours; ** ER-positive tumours

operative chemotherapy [7] and the other assessed 5 years of tamoxifen treatment [8] (Table 4). All of these trials compared a control versus a treatment group. Although inclusion criteria, type and duration of adjuvant treatment were different, the clinical outcome, with a median follow-up of 3-4 years, was quite similar. Toxic effects were generally at an acceptable level in all studies. In all 4 studies, a statistically significant improvement was found for disease-free survival but not for overall survival.

Long-term follow-up is required before final conclusions may be drawn from the current findings; moreover, additional randomised trials that include "high-risk" node-negative tumours in all age groups of patients need to be conducted.

## New Trial Designs in Node-Negative Tumours

Benefit from systemic adjuvant therapy with cytostatic combinations as well as endocrine (tamoxifen) treatment has been demonstrated. The first adjuvant randomised trials in operable breast cancer compared the effects of ovarian ablation with those of no further treatment after mastectomy [9-11].

Endocrine manipulation, which is generally possible by irradiation, surgery or medical ablation as well as by cytotoxic treatment, may result in a prognostic benefit. However, adjuvant hormonal treatment for premenopausal patients, or even its use in different age groups and for groups with different hormone receptor status, is controversial. Data from the German Adjuvant Breast Cancer Group (GABG) Trial I [12] demonstrated significant benefit for premenopausal patients treated with 6 cycles of CMF in terms of disease-free survival (DFS) and overall survival (OS) with 1-3 positive nodes and hormone receptor-positive tumours and for postmenopausal patients treated with tamoxifen for 2 years (DFS). In most trials, ovarian suppression (ovarian ablation or cytotoxically-induced amenorrhoea) resulted in some benefit for young (premenopausal) women [4,10,11,13,14].

Major questions concerning appropriate adjuvant treatment for node-negative tumours must be answered for the future:

1. Who are candidates for no adjuvant treatment?

2. Who are candidates for adjuvant systemic cytotoxic treatment, endocrine treatment or both modalities?
3. Who are candidates for adjuvant radiotherapy with or without systemic therapy for breast-conserving surgical treatment?

Moreover, optimal drug combinations, drug doses, optimal duration of therapies, optimal treatment intervals and sequences must be established in new trials.

Tables 5 and 6 show new international and German (GABG IV BMFT IV) study designs for different tumour and patient subsets. These new designs focus mainly on endocrine (tamoxifen or ovarian ablation) versus cytotoxic regimens. Ovarian ablation is achieved by medical castration produced by a GnRH-depot analogue formulation (Zoladex). Zoladex yielded objective response rates in more than 40% of premenopausal metastatic

**Table 5.** New international adjuvant studies in node-negative breast cancer

*Primary breast cancer N⁻*

| **Study** | **Subgroups** | **Randomisation** |
|---|---|---|
| IBCSG Trial V | premenopausal + perimenopausal | control vs Zoladex 2 yrs vs CMF x 6 vs CMF x 6 + Zoladex 1.5 years |
| IBCSG Trial IX | postmenopausal | Tam vs CMF Tam |
| NSABP B-19 | ER- | MF vs CMF |
| NSABP B-20 | ER+ | Tam vs MFT vs CMFT |
| Intergroup Trial | ER? | CAF ± T vs CMF ± T |
| CRC Trial | N± * < 50 years | control vs Tam 2 years vs Zoladex vs Zoladex+Tam |

* periop. CMF allowed; T = Tam

**Table 6.** New German (united GABG and BMFT trial group) adjuvant studies in node-negative breast cancer

*Primary breast cancer N± (n: 0-9 involved)*

| **Study** | | **Subgroups** ER/PR; menopausal status | **Randomisation** |
|---|---|---|---|
| A) T ≤ 3cm $G_1$ - $2_a$ | + | premenopausal postmenopausal | control vs RT |
| B) | + | premenopausal | CMF x 6 vs Zoladex 2 years |
| C) | + | postmenopausal | Tam 2 years vs Tam 2 years --> AR 3 years |
| D) | - | premenopausal/ postmenopausal | CMF x 6 vs CMF x 6 + hormonal replacement |

T > 3 cm: mod. rad. mastectomy

T = primary tumour site; G = grading; RT = radiotherapy; AR = aromatase inhibitor

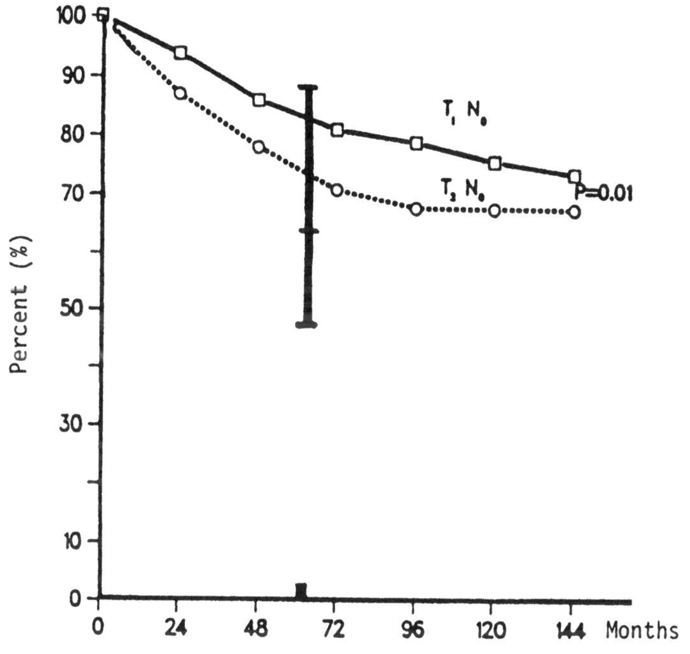


**Fig. 1.** Relapse-free survival data of node-negative breast cancer by axillary lymph nodes and primary tumour size in the Natural History Data Base [20] - Comparison with the range of reported 5-year data of control arms in adjuvant trials

breast cancer patients [15]. The advantages of such GnRH analogues are the reversibility of ovarian ablation after cessation of administration of this drug, as well as its possible direct effect on the tumour cells [16]. In some international trials, also node-positive tumours, and in the German trials all node-negative and node-positive tumours with up to 9 involved nodes are included. Primary tumour size is the most important factor in the surgical decision-making for modified mastectomy or breast-conserving management. It is in these cases that an impact from adjuvant radiotherapy in node-negative, grade 1-2a tumours should be proven.

It is important to obtain further information on the role of less aggressive primary surgery and radiotherapy combined with systemic treatment modalities, because all data have thus far been derived from patients who underwent radical or modified radical mastectomy.

## Node-Negative Tumours: Prognosis and Accurate Assessment of Nodal Status

The only prognostic factor that has proven to be predictive of recurrence or mortality is axillary lymph-node status [17,18]. However, 5-year relapse-free survival data from the Natural History Data Base [19] vary, also with tumour size.

A comparison of 5-year relapse-free survival rates also demonstrates that control groups in surgery and adjuvant treatment trials differ within a range of 93-45% (Fig. 1). Studies that focus on the treatment of node-negative breast cancer necessarily make a selection among patients with primary breast cancer, and results may therefore be biased by various factors.

Two questions must be answered for an accurate identification of lymph-node negative or "low-risk" status:

1. What staging procedures should be used to ensure that a patient's nodal status is negative?
2. Does, for instance, primary (neo-adjuvant) systemic treatment influence nodal status?

At present, only on the basis of surgical clearance and thorough histological examination can information about the involvement of the axilla be obtained and correct staging be performed. The axilla is divided into 3 levels (I,II,III). Data on "skip" metastases [20,21] show that clearance and information on levels I and II are sufficient for ascertaining whether a tumour is node negative. In our surgical series, before 1978, the mean num-

**Table 10.** Risk-benefit analysis for systemic adjuvant therapy in operable breast cancer

| | CHT | HT (Tam/GnRH/AR) |
|---|---|---|
| **Interaction with RT:** | (+) | ? |
| **Short-term toxicity:** | | |
| Alopecia, vomiting | +++ | (-) |
| hot flushes | (-) | + |
| Thrombosis/embolism | + | (-) |
| **Long-term toxicity:** | | |
| Leukaemia | (+) | - |
| Endometrium cancer | - | + |
| Osteoporosis | ? | (+) |
| **Protection against:** | | |
| Osteoporosis/atherosclerosis | - | +/- |
| Breast cancer | - | (+) |
| **Economic costs:** | + | ++ |

RT = radiotherapy; CHT = chemotherapy
HT = endocrine therapy

from all the participating centres more consistent, also for the purpose of reliable interstudy comparisons.

## Risk-Benefit Analyses

The large, recently published, adjuvant trials have demonstrated benefit only in terms of disease-free survival, which is of great importance for an improvement in the quality of life of these women. The question whether longer disease-free survival also results in prolongation of survival, is still unanswered.
Table 10 gives a summary of proven and possible toxicities together with economic costs. It is clear that the short-term toxic effects of chemotherapy are more substantial than those of endocrine treatment. However, supportive care clearly is of value. In contrast, data on long-term toxicities as well as protection against, for instance, contralateral breast cancer, are not available. Economic costs are usually higher for endocrine manipulations than, for example, for the CMF regimen. New proposals for individual risk-benefit analyses have been made [24]. Assessment of toxicity from adjuvant treatment and during long-term follow-up in relation to outcome is an essential component of adjuvant therapy strategies for node-negative breast cancer, which usually has a better prognosis than node-positive tumours.

## Conclusions

For medical reasons, improvement of disease-free survival may be of benefit in operable breast cancer. However, this must be considered in relation to the "costs" to the patient. In this case, adjuvant endocrine treatment seems to be more appropriate. However, the primary aim of systemic adjuvant treatment in the cure of women with operable breast cancer may be attainable only by cytotoxic drugs. To date, "low-risk" and "high-risk" situations have not been established in node-negative breast cancer. Further direct comparisons of adjuvant cytotoxic and endocrine treatment in prospectively defined subsets of breast cancer patients are needed. No recommendation of a standard treatment for node-negative breast cancer can be made at present on the basis of data from randomised trials. Therefore, adjuvant systemic therapy outside of clinical trials is unjustified in node-negative breast cancer.

## REFERENCES


1 Early Breast Cancer Trialists Collaborative Group: The effects of adjuvant tamoxifen and of cytotoxic therapy on mortality in early breast cancer: An overview of 61 randomized trials among 28,896 women. N Engl J Med 1988 (319):1681-1692

2 Glick JH: Closing summary and outlook. In: Senn HJ, Goldhirsch A, Gelber RD, Osterwalder B (eds): Adjuvant Therapy of Primary Breast Cancer. Recent Results in Cancer Research. Springer, Berlin 1989 pp 283-292

3 Bonadonna G: Conceptual and practical advances in the management of breast cancer: The 20th Annual Karnofsky Award Lecture. J Clin Oncol 1989 (10):1380-1397

4 Henderson IC: Adjuvant systemic therapy: State of the art, 1989. 11th San Antonio Breast Cancer Symposium Lecture. Breast Cancer Res Treatm 1989 (14):3-22

5 Fisher B, Redmond C, Dimitrov NV et al: A randomized clinical trial evaluating sequential methotrexate and fluorouracil in the treatment of patients with node-negative breast cancer who have estrogen-receptor-negative tumors. N Engl J Med 1989 (320):473 478

6 Mansour EG, Gray R, Shatila AH et al: Efficacy of adjuvant chemotherapy in high-risk node-negative breast cancer: an intergroup study. N Engl J Med. 1989 (320):485-490

7 Ludwig Breast Cancer Study Group: Prolonged disease-free survival after one course of perioperative adjuvant chemotherapy for node-negative breast cancer. N Engl J Med 1989 (320): 491-496

8 Fisher B, Constantino J, Redmond C, et al: A randomized clinical trial evaluating tamoxifen in the treatment of patients with node-negative breast cancer who have estrogen-receptor-positive tumors. N Engl J Med 1989 (320):479-484

9 Bryant AJ, Weir JA: Prophylactic oophorectomy in operable instances of carcinoma of the breast. Surg Gynecol Obstet 1981 (153):660-664

10 Cole MP: Prophylactic compared with therapeutic x-ray artifical menopause. 2nd Tenovus Workshop of Breast Cancer, 1970 pp 2-11

11 Ravdin RG, Lewison EF, Slack NH et al: Results of a clinical trial concerning the worth of prophylactic oophorectomy for breast carcinoma. Surg Gynecol Obstet 1970 (31):1055-1064

12 Kaufmann M, Jonat W, Abel U: Adjuvant chemo- and endocrine therapy alone or in combination in premenopausal patients (GABG Trial I). In: Senn HJ, Goldhirsch A, Gelber RD, Osterwalder B (eds): Adjuvant Therapy of Primary Breast Cancer. Recent Results in Cancer Research. Springer, Berlin 1989 pp 118-125

13 Meakin JW, Allt WEC, Beale FA et al: Ovarian irradiation and prednisone following surgery and radiotherapy for carcinoma of the breast. Breast Cancer Res Treat 1983 (3 supp):45-48

14 Meakin JW, Allt WEC, Beale FA et al: Ovarian irradiation and prednisone therapy following surgery and radiotherapy for carcinoma of the breast. Can Med Assoc J 1979 (120):1221-1228

15 Kaufmann M, Jonat W, Kleeberg U, Eiermann W, Jänicke F, Hilfrich J, Kreienberg R, Albrecht M, Weitzel HK, Schmid H, Strunz P, Schachner-Wünschmann E, Bastert G, Maass H, for the German Zoladex Trial Group: Goserelin, a depot gonadotrophin-releasing hormone agonist in the treatment of premenopausal patients with metastatic breast cancer: J Clin Oncol 1989 (7):1113-1119

16 Kiesel L, Kaufmann M, Haeseler F, Klinga K, von Holst T, Schmidt W, Runnebaum B: GnRH-Rezeptoren im menschlichen Mammakarzinomgewebe: Geburts u Frauenheilk 1988 (48): 420-424

17 Carter CL, Allen, Henson DE: Relation of tumor size, lymph node status, and survival in 24740 breast cancer cases. Cancer 1989 (63):181-187

18 Müller A, Kubli F, Tschahargane C, Schindler E, Kaufmann M.: Bedeutung der histologischen Aufarbeitung der Axilla beim Staging des invasiven Mammakarzinoms, In: Hermanek P (ed) Bedeutung des TNM-Systems für die klinische Onkologie. Zuckschwerdt, München, Bern, Wien 1986 pp 54-59

19 Moon E, Jones E, Tong T, Serokman R, Bonadonna G, Veronesi U, Vaugussa P, Powles TJ, Buzdar A, Montague E: Development of a natural history data base of breast cancer studies: In: Salmon SE (ed) Adjuvant Therapy of Cancer. Grune & Stratton, Orlando 1987 pp 227-233

20 Kubli F, Müller A, Kaufmann M: Die axilläre Lymphonodektomie in der Therapieplanung beim invasiven Mammakarzinom: In: Hepp H, Scheidel P, Monaghan JM (eds): Lymphonodektomie in der gynäkologischen Onkologie. Urban & Schwarzenburg, München, Wien, Baltimore 1988 pp 115-124

21 Rosen P, Lesser M, Kinne D, Beattie E: Discontinous or "skip" metastases in breast cancer: Analysis of 1228 axillary dissections. Ann Surg 1983 (197):276

22 Jarasch ED, Nagle R, Kaufmann M, Maurer C, Böcker WJ: Differential diagnosis of benign epithelial proliferations and carcinomas of the breast using antibodies to cytokeratins. Hum Pathol 1988 (19):276-289

23 Kaufmann M, Feichter GE, Nhila A, Klinga K, Abel U: Flowzytophotometrische Parameter, Hormonrezeptoren und axillärer Lymphknotenstatus als Prognosefaktoren beim primären Mammakarzinom. Geburtsh u Frauenheilk 1988 (48):705-709

24 Goldhirsch A, Gelber RD, Simes RJ, et al, For the Ludwig Breast Cancer Study Group: Costs and benefits of adjuvant therapy in breast cancer: A quality adjusted survival analysis. J Clin Oncol 1989 (7):36-44

25 Nissen-Meyer R, Host H, Kjellgren K, Mansson B, Norin T: Neoadjuvant chemotherapy in breast cancer: As single perioperative treatment and with supplementary long-term chemotherapy. In: Salmon SE (ed) Adjuvant Therapy of Cancer. Grune & Stratton, Orlando 1987 pp 253-261

26 Senn HJ, Barett-Mahler R, for the OSAKO and SAKK Groups: Update of Swiss adjuvant trials with LMF and CMF in operable breast cancer. In: Salmon SE (ed) Adjuvant Therapy of Cancer. Grune & Stratton, Orlando 1987 pp 243-252
27 Morrison JM, Howell A, Grieve RJ, Monypenny IJ, Walter R, Kelly KA, Waterhouse JA: The West Midlands Oncology Association trials of adjuvant chemotherapy for operable breast cancer. In: Salmon SE (ed) Adjuvant Therapy of Cancer. Grune & Stratton, Orlando 1987 pp 311-318
28 Jakesz R, Kolb R, Reiner G, Schemper M, Rainer H, Dittrich C, Reiner A: Adjuvant chemotherapy in node-negative breast cancer patients. In: Salmon SE (ed) Adjuvant Therapy of Cancer. Grune & Stratton, Orlando 1987 pp 223-231
29 Scottish Cancer Trials Office: Adjuvant tamoxifen in the management of operable breast cancer: The Scottish Trial. Lancet 1987 (ii):171-175
30 Nolvadex Adjuvant Trial Organisation: Controlled trial of tamoxifen as a single adjuvant agent in the management of early breast cancer. Br J Cancer 1988 (57):608-611
31 CRC Adjuvant Breast Trial Working Party: Cyclophosphamide and tamoxifen as adjuvant therapies in the management of breast cancer. Br J Cancer 1988 (57):604-607
32 Fornander T, Cedermark B, Mattson A et al: Adjuvant tamoxifen in early breast cancer: Occurence of new primary cancers. Lancet 1989 (i):117-120

# Adjuvant Chemotherapy in Premenopausal Breast Cancer Patients is Effective by Means Other than Ovarian Function Suppression

A. Goldhirsch [1], R.D. Gelber [2] and M. Castiglione [3],
for The International Breast Cancer Study Group (formerly Ludwig Group)

1 Division of Oncology, Ospedale San Giovanni, Bellinzona, and Ospedale Civico, Lugano, Switzerland
2 Harvard Medical School, Harvard School of Public Health and Dana-Farber Cancer Institute, Boston, MA, U.S.A.
3 Institute of Medical Oncology, Inselspital, University of Bern, Bern, Switzerland

## Summary

In order further to clarify the role of endocrine mechanisms mediating the effect of adjuvant systemic therapy in patients with operable breast cancer, we analysed the incidence of amenorrhoea and its association with outcome in a cohort of 1127 premenopausal women included in a randomised trial. There were 4 distinct subpopulations defined by nodal status and therapy: in a group with node-negative disease (552 patients), one course of cytotoxic drugs was compared to no adjuvant chemotherapy. In a group with metastatic nodes (575 patients), a single course of cytotoxic therapy was compared with a prolonged treatment (6 or 7 courses). Amenorrhoea was defined as having no menstrual bleeding for a 3-month interval within the first 9 months after surgery. Amenorrhoea was observed in 21% of the 199 patients with N-negative breast cancer who received no adjuvant therapy, in 31% of the 353 N-negative patients who had a single course of cytotoxic therapy and in 31% of the 188 patients with N-positive disease who had the same short-duration therapy as compared to 68% of the 387 patients who had a prolonged adjuvant therapy. Amenorrhoea was associated with a prolonged disease-free survival (DFS) only in the patients with prolonged cytotoxic therapy: 4-year DFS % (+ s.e.) was 68% + 3% vs 61% + 5%, for the amenorrhoea and the no-amenorrhoea groups, respectively ($p=0.05$). On the other hand, the comparison between the effects of prolonged therapy upon outcome versus the short perioperative course (the direct comparison of the trial carried out within the node-positive population) showed a much larger treatment effect. The 4-year DFS% was 66% as compared to 38% ($p<0.0001$).

We conclude that cytotoxic-induced amenorrhoea is associated with a better outcome, but that this effect is difficult to observe due to the non cytotoxic-induced amenorrhoea rate, which is substantial in a patient population with breast cancer. The influence of amenorrhoea upon outcome is of small magnitude and it is unlikely that the effect of cytotoxics to reduce relapse and mortality rates in premenopausal women with breast cancer is primarily due to an ovarian suppression-mediated mechanism.

## Introduction

Since the time when the natural history of the disease was first understood, averting relapse from breast cancer has been a major concern for clinicians. Endocrine ablative therapy was found to induce remissions in locally advanced disease long before the endocrine mechanisms which lead to such a response were even suspected [1]. It is not surprising that one of the first reasonably controlled trials of cancer therapy was an early study in the mid forties by Paterson et al.

at the Christie Hospital in Manchester. By the early seventies, before the current hypothesis on the physiopathology of relapse was formulated, 9 randomised trials had investigated the role of ovarian ablation in early breast cancer [2]. These were typically small studies and did not show differences of relevant or significant magnitude during the first decade of follow up. It has been accepted since the mid seventies that micrometastatic disease already present at diagnosis will eventually cause symptomatic relapse in many patients [3]. Two additional studies were initiated after that time to assess the role of ovarian ablation added to chemotherapy. Summing up all these trials of ovarian ablation (either surgical or radiation-induced), 1280 patients less than 50 years of age and 1023 women 50 years old or older were included. Despite the non availability of some follow-up data, the Early Breast Cancer Trialists Collaborative Group performed an overview of these trials which estimated the magnitude of the reduction in the odds of death to be 22%±10% and 11%±9% among the younger and the older subpopulations, respectively [4].

That adjuvant systemic chemotherapy is effective in reducing relapse and early mortality has recently been shown by the meta-analysis performed upon all available results from randomised trials by the same Collaborative Group [4]. The beneficial effect of adjuvant prolonged multidrug chemotherapy in reducing relapse and mortality has been observed in premenopausal patients already early during follow up [2]. Initial investigations aimed to correlate this effect upon outcome with the amenorrhoea observed in a substantial proportion of the patients were performed on a small number of women (76 patients treated with melphalan alone and 20 patients treated with melphalan and 5-fluorouracil) included in two National Surgical Adjuvant Breast and Bowel Project (NSABP) studies [5], and in the Milan study (78 patients) [6]. These investigations yielded a lack of relationship between amenorrhoea and treatment effect. Additional investigations were conducted for 1839 patients included in Ludwig Trial I [7], the Eastern Cooperative Oncology Group (ECOG) study [8], the Guy's Hospital study [9], and the Danish Breast Cancer Study Group's trial [10]. The results of these analyses showed some association between the cessation of menstrual cycle and outcome. The effects of amenorrhoea were also confounded with the oestrogen receptor content of the primary tumour [6,8]: the effect of amenorrhoea was seen almost exclusively in the subpopulation of patients with positive oestrogen receptors. These observations led to the speculation that adjuvant cytotoxic therapy is effective only because it causes a chemical ovarian function suppression [8]. The fact that adjuvant cytotoxic therapy is also effective in patients with tumours having no oestrogen receptors [11], and the observation of an early onset of its effects (as opposed to the delayed effect of treatment observed in all trials with surgical or radiation-induced ovarian ablation), have been used as arguments against a major role of an endocrine mechanism. Very recently some trials have been initiated to directly compare the effects of adjuvant chemotherapy and ovarian ablation. The results of these trials will not be available for several years. In the meantime, the search for indirect evidence which might explain the mechanism of action of adjuvant systemic chemotherapy is warranted. An extensive analysis of a premenopausal patient population with breast cancer who received no cytotoxic therapy, a short course of treatment or a prolonged chemotherapy, and for which the menstrual data were known, has not yet been attempted and is the subject of this report.

## Methods

From November 1981 to December 1985, 2628 patients with breast cancer or candidates for a surgical procedure to ascertain the presence of breast cancer were randomly assigned to receive either perioperative combination chemotherapy (to be started within 36 hours of mastectomy), or no perioperative chemotherapy (Table 1). Patients classified as having a node-negative disease received no additional adjuvant therapy. The patients found to have metastatic lymph nodes were treated according to initial assignment with no additional chemotherapy (a perioperative therapy alone group), or with a conventionally-timed chemotherapy regimen

**Table 1.** Study design and treatment regimens for premenopausal patients in international Trial V

| | | Perioperative period (≤ 36 hrs) | Commencing 25-36 days postoperative if N- | if N+ |
|---|---|---|---|---|
| R | --> | PeCT | - | - |
| A | | | | |
| N | --> | PeCT | - | CMFpx6 |
| D | | | | |
| O | --> | No PeCT | - | CMFpx6 |
| M | | | | |

PeCT: Perioperative Therapy (started within 36 hours after surgery):
a single course of i.v. CMF: cyclophosphamide 400 mg/m$^2$, methotrexate 40 mg/m$^2$, 5-fluorouracil 600 mg/m$^2$ all i.v. days 1 and 8; leucovorin 15 mg i.v. on day 2 and orally on day 9 (for details see references 12,13)

CMFp: C = cyclophosphamide 100 mg/m$^2$ orally days 1-14
MF = methotrexate and 5-fluorouracil: as above
p = prednisone 7.5 mg daily continuously q 28 days for 6 courses

The CMFpx6 was commenced either on day 29 of the PeCT cycle (if assigned) or between days 25-36 after mastectomy for patients who had no PeCT

which consisted of 6 courses as specified in Table 1.

The eligibility and evaluability of the patients were extensively published [12,13]. Results related to treatment effects in both, node-positive and node-negative, populations at a median observation time of 42 months were reported.

1127 premenopausal women who had their last normal menstrual period within 6 months before mastectomy were evaluable for the analysis of treatment effects according to observed amenorrhoea. Amenorrhoea was defined as having had no menstrual bleeding for at least a 3-month interval within the first 9 months after definitive surgery for breast cancer. The causes for ineligibility for this specific analysis are described in Table 2. A "landmark analysis" [14] excluding all patients who relapsed within the first 9 months was performed in order to avoid bias. In fact, the analysis of disease-free survival by amenorrhoea might be biased because of the reduced possibility for patients who relapsed within the first 9 months to develop amenorrhoea. The "landmark analysis" in which all these patients are excluded removes this misclassification due to relapse-dependent condition.

**Table 2.** Evaluability of premenopausal patients for analysis on effects of amenorrhoea (% are in parentheses)

| | N- No PeCT | N- PeCT | N+ PeCT alone | N+ CMFpx6 (±PeCT) |
|---|---|---|---|---|
| Total Eligible | 238 | 454 | 244 | 471 |
| Evaluable | 199 (84) | 353 (78) | 188 (77) | 387 (82) |
| Non-evaluable | | | | |
| Reasons: | | | | |
| Hysterectomy | 21 (9) | 54 (12) | 34 (14) | 53 (11) |
| Perimenopausal | 13 (5) | 25 ( 6) | 18 ( 7) | 17 ( 4) |
| No Chemotherapy | -- | -- | -- | 9 (2) |
| > 1 course | -- | 2 (<1) | -- | -- |
| Lack of Information | 5 (2) | 20 ( 4) | 4 ( 2) | 5 (1) |

**Table 6.** Estimated 4-year disease-free survival percentages (±s.e.) according to amenorrhoea status excluding patients who relapse whithin 9 months after surgery (LANDMARK ANALYSIS) (numbers of patients in parentheses)

| | N- No PeCT | N- PeCT | N+ PeCT alone | N+ CMFpx6 (±PeCT) |
|---|---|---|---|---|
| TOTAL PATIENTS | 75± 3 (189) | 79± 2 (344) | 46± 5 (156) | 68± 3 (373) |
| Amenorrhoea | 78± 7 ( 39) | 82± 4 (107) | 45± 8 ( 47) | 70± 3 (254) |
| No Amenorrhoea | 75± 4 (150) | 78± 3 (237) | 46± 5 (109) | 63± 5 (119) |
| p-value | 0.93 | 0.09 | 0.97 | 0.05 |
| AGE | | | | |
| ≤ 40 | | | | |
| Amenorrhoea | 67±21 ( 3) | 88±12 ( 8) | 33±19 ( 6) | 66±10 (30) |
| No Amenorrhoea | 71± 8 (45) | 73± 6 (74) | 48± 9 (38) | 62± 6 (67) |
| p-value | 0.63 | 0.34 | 0.13 | 0.69 |
| ≥ 40 | | | | |
| Amenorrhoea | 79± 7 ( 36) | 82± 5 ( 99) | 47± 9 (41) | 71± 3 (224) |
| No Amenorrhoea | 76± 5 (105) | 81± 3 (163) | 45± 7 (71) | 66± 7 ( 52) |
| p-value | 0.82 | 0.33 | 0.66 | 0.11 |
| ER Status | | | | |
| ER+ | | | | |
| Amenorrhoea | 74±12 (19) | 81± 6 (52) | 38± 11 (25) | 74± 4 (135) |
| No Amenorrhoea | 72± 6 (66) | 76± 5 (92) | 51± 8 (55) | 68± 7 ( 59) |
| p-value | 0.68 | 0.25 | 0.44 | 0.09 |
| ER- | | | | |
| Amenorrhoea | 82±12 (11) | 83± 8 ( 29) | 53±15 (15) | 60± 6 ( 94) |
| No Amenorrhoea | 77± 6 (57) | 80± 5 (101) | 30± 8 (36) | 59± 8 ( 40) |
| p-value | 0.87 | 0.83 | 0.29 | 0.69 |
| ER unknown | | | | |
| Amenorrhoea | 76±15 ( 9) | 86± 8 (26) | 57±19 ( 7) | 90± 7 (25) |
| No Amenorrhoea | 77± 9 (27) | 76± 7 (44) | 58±12 (18) | 51±17 (20) |
| p-value | 0.84 | 0.09 | 0.95 | 0.02 |

Amenorrhoea was not associated with improved disease-free survival for either the node-negative patients, or the node-positive patients who received a single cycle of chemotherapy (Table 5). The apparently worse outcome for patients in the latter group who developed amenorrhoea can be attributed to the misclassification bias that was corrected in the "landmark analysis" shown in Table 6.

The association of induced amenorrhoea with improved disease-free survival for node-positive patients who received prolonged chemotherapy remained statistically significant in the "landmark analysis" (Table 6).

The comparison of disease-free survival between the treatment groups for node-positive patients favoured the prolonged chemotherapy regimen (66% versus 38%; p<0.0001; Fig. 2 and Table 5). This treatment effect difference was equally seen for both the younger patients (59% versus 33%; p<0.0001) and the older patients (68% versus 40%; p<0.0001).

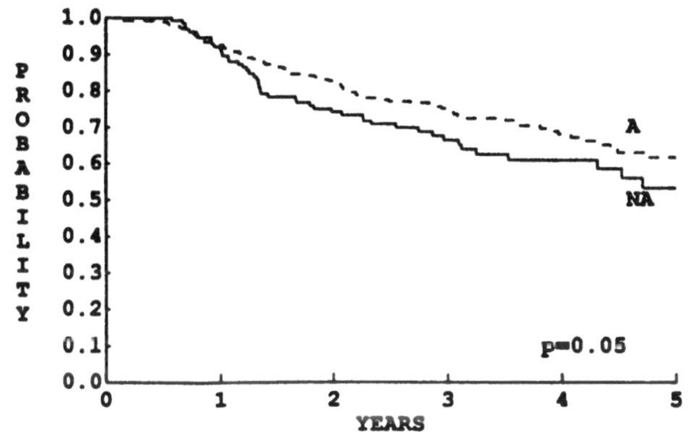


At Risk

| | | | | | | |
|---|---|---|---|---|---|---|
| A | 263 | 243 | 210 | 148 | 84 | 36 |
| NA | 124 | 113 | 89 | 57 | 31 | 19 |

**Fig. 1.** Disease-free survival according to amenorrhoea status for 387 premenopausal women with axillary node involvement who received prolonged cytotoxic treatment (48 months median follow up)
A denotes amenorrhoea, NA denotes no amenorrhoea

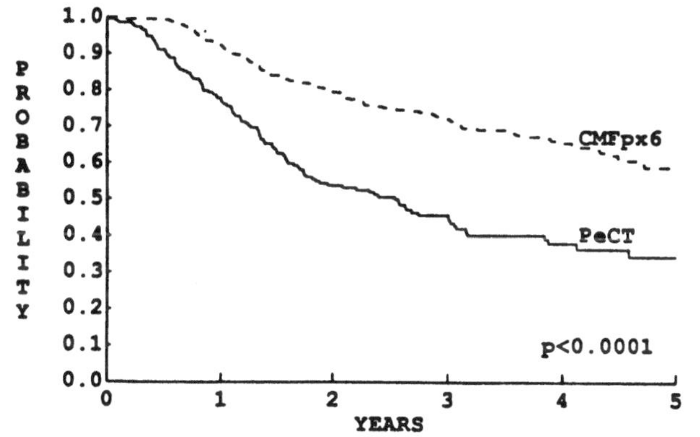


At Risk

| | | | | | | |
|---|---|---|---|---|---|---|
| CMFpx6 | 387 | 356 | 299 | 205 | 115 | 55 |
| PeCT | 188 | 144 | 93 | 61 | 34 | 11 |

**Fig. 2.** Disease-free survival according to treatment group for 575 premenopausal women with axillary node involvement (48 months median follow up)
PeCT denotes perioperative chemotherapy alone, CMFpx6 denotes prolonged cytotoxic treatment

## Discussion

Endocrine ablative therapy has been shown to have a significant effect upon outcome of premenopausal breast cancer patients. Recently, even the antioestrogen agent, tamoxifen, has been demonstrated to improve disease-free survival for patients with node-negative breast cancer and oestrogen receptor-positive primaries [18]. The exact role of adjuvant ablative endocrine therapy alone has not completely been elucidated for the young population of breast cancer patients. This fact has been mainly due to the larger therapeutic effect of adjuvant chemotherapy upon outcome [3]. The indirect comparisons between more recently conducted chemotherapy trials and older ovarian ablation studies convinced many that for premenopausal women cytotoxics represent a more effective adjuvant regimen. This has also been the case for the indirect comparison between results of cytotoxics and adjuvant tamoxifen [2]. In fact, only one trial has been published which directly compared tamoxifen with a cyclophosphamide, methotrexate, 5-fluorouracil combination chemotherapy in 120 premenopausal women with both, oestrogen or progesterone-positive primaries and one to three involved axillary nodes [19].This trial demonstrated a significant advantage in terms of disease-free survival for the patients who received CMF adjuvant therapy. The entire issue obviously awaits confirmation.

The role of cytotoxics-induced amenorrhoea has been questioned in retrospective analyses of 6 series on 2013 patients, and has been found to relate to outcome in 896 patients treated with CMF (+/- prednisone high dose +/- tamoxifen) [7,8,9] and in 424 patients treated with cyclophosphamide alone [10]. No association with outcome was reported for patients treated with melphalan alone or with melphalan and 5-fluorouracil [5] or with CMF (+/- low-dose prednisone) [6,7,10].

In Ludwig Trial I, 399 of the 491 pre- and perimenopausal patients with node-positive breast cancer were evaluable for the effects of chemotherapy-induced amenorrhoea upon treatment outcome. In this trial, premenopausal patients with a relatively "good prognosis" (1-3 axillary nodes involved) were randomised to receive 12 courses of a cyclophosphamide, methotrexate, 5-fluorouracil (CMF) combination therapy with or without low-dose prednisone [7]. Induced amenorrhoea was associated with a longer disease-free survival for younger patients (age 39 years or less), patients who received lower

CMF doses (<80% of the average dose specified in the protocol) and patients with ER-positive primaries. The difference was also only observed in the CMF treatment group (i.e., without prednisone therapy).
A similar analysis for the premenopausal cohort of Trial V, including a large group of patients who received cytotoxic therapies of different durations, provided the following information. A shorter duration of therapy was always related to a lower incidence of amenorrhoea and this amenorrhoea was not associated with outcome. The "spontaneous amenorrhoea rate" ( i.e., in the group which received no adjuvant chemotherapy after mastectomy) was found to be 21% in our selected population, 6% in the younger age group and 26% in the group of 40 years old or more. One single cycle of cytotoxic drugs (with cyclophosphamide given i.v., a route of administration usually associated with less ovarian failures even if administered for longer duration) was sufficient to increase the amenorrhoea rates to 10% in the younger patients and 33% for the older cohort. Six or 7 courses of chemotherapy (with cyclophosphamide administered orally for 14 days each course, a treatment known to be associated with more ovarian function suppression than the one with cyclophosphamide given i.v.) yielded a larger proportion of patients who ceased menses: 33% and 81%, respectively. In Trial I the amenorrhoea rates after **12 courses** of the same chemotherapy for the same age groups were 61% and 95%, respectively. Due to these distributions, it is clear that in Trial I effects of amenorrhoea on outcome, if they exist, were demonstrable exclusively in the younger patients.
In Trial V, a significantly lower incidence of amenorrhoea was obtained in the younger age group for which no association was observed between cessation of menses and outcome. This might be due to the fact that on the one hand, even in the younger group, some patients were predicted to lose ovarian endocrine activity, as demonstrated from the no-adjuvant group. On the other hand, only 33% of the patients (34 out of 103) in this group had amenorrhoea induced by the prolonged treatment and 56% of these resumed menses within 15 months (19 patients). Thus, too few young patients might have experienced treatment-induced amenorrhoea which was sufficient to produce some effect upon outcome.
In order to avoid a bias which relates to the dependence between observation time and the time elapsed until ovarian function suppression, a "landmark" analysis was performed. This excluded all patients who relapsed within the 9-month time period in which the observation of suppression of menses had to be made. The association between better prognosis and induced amenorrhoea was similar to the analysis done by including all patients in the analysis (Tables 5 and 6).
Evidence exists, even if indirect, that amenorrhoea is beneficial for premenopausal patients. It is unlikely that the entire effect of cytotoxic adjuvant therapy is mediated by such an endocrine manipulation, however, because the treatment effects of chemotherapy are much larger than the outcome differences observed for patients who do or do not have amenorrhoea. For our cohort of patients with node-positive breast cancer, the single cycle of perioperative chemotherapy was associated with a 4-year disease-free survival of 38% compared with 66% for patients who received the prolonged cytotoxic regimen. This difference represents the chemotherapy effect. Although differences according to amenorrhoea status were statistically significant in the group that was treated with a prolonged regimen, the 4-year disease-free survival percentages were 61% compared to 68%. This smaller difference might be ascribed to the endocrine effect of ovarian function suppression.
Even more striking is the contrast between the chemotherapy effect and the amenorrhoea effect in the younger population. For patients younger than 40 years of age the difference in favour of prolonged chemotherapy compared with the single course of treatment was highly significant (4-year DFS%=59% versus 33%; $p<0.0001$). The presence of amenorrhoea in this cohort did not provide any improvement in outcome for either treatment regimen.
It remains to be determined to what extent the mechanism of action of chemotherapy in premenopausal patients is related to endocrine effects. It is possible that the chemotherapy-induced amenorrhoea is a marker for a more efficient tumour cell kill by

the cytotoxics. The role of induced amenorrhoea might best be elucidated by a randomised trial allocating patients to surgical or LH-RH analogue induced castration following the administration of chemotherapy.
Such a trial has just been initiated by the International Breast Cancer Study Group (Trial VIII) for node-negative premenopausal women. Patients are randomised to receive either CMF chemotherapy, **or** the same chemotherapy followed by the LH-RH analogue Zoladex **or** Zoladex alone **or** no adjuvant therapy. An accurate monthly recording of menstrual history is planned for patients in Trial VIII which will provide prospectively collected data on the importance of ovarian function suppression as a mechanism for adjuvant chemotherapy effectiveness.

## Acknowledgement

We thank all the patients, physicians, nurses and data managers who participate in the International Breast Cancer Study Group trials. We also gratefully acknowledge the support for central coordination, data management and statistics provided by the Swiss Cancer League, Cancer League of Ticino, Swiss Group for Clinical Cancer Research, Australia - New Zealand Breast Cancer Study Group, and Frontier Science & Technology Research Foundation.

## REFERENCES


1 Beatson GT: On the treatment of inoperable cases of carcinoma of the mammae: suggestions for a new method of treatment with illustrative cases. Lancet 1896 (ii):104-107

2 Goldhirsch A, Gelber RD, Mouridsen H: Adjuvant chemotherapy in premenopausal patients: a more complicated form of oophorectomy? In: Cavalli F (ed) Endocrine Therapy for Breast Cancer II. European School of Oncology Monographs. Springer Verlag, Berlin 1987 pp 11-19

3 Henderson IC, Canellos GP: Cancer of the breast: the past decade. N Engl J Med 1980 (302):17-30

4 Early Breast Cancer Trialists' Collaborative Group: Effects of adjuvant tamoxifen and of cytotoxic therapy on mortality in early breast cancer. An overview of 61 randomized trials among 28,896 women. N Engl J Med 1988 (319):1681-1692

5 Fisher B, Sherman B, Rockette H et al: L-phenylalanine mustard (L-PAM) in the management of premenopausal patients with primary breast cancer: lack of association of DFS with depression of ovarian function. Cancer 1979 (44):847-857

6 Bonadonna G, Valagussa P, Rossi A et al: Ten-year experience with CMF-based adjuvant chemotherapy in resectable breast cancer. Breast Cancer Res Treat 1985 (5):95-115

7 Ludwig Breast Cancer Study Group: A randomized trial of adjuvant combination chemotherapy with or without prednisone in premenopausal breast cancer patients with metastases in one to three axillary lymph nodes. Cancer Res 1985 (45):4454-4459

8 Tormey DC: Adjuvant systemic therapy in postoperative node+ patients with breast carcinoma: the CALGB trial and the ECOG premenopausal trial. In Senn HJ (ed) Recent Results in Cancer Research. Adjuvant Chemotherapy of Breast Cancer. Springer Verlag, Heidelberg-Berlin 1984 pp 155-165

9 Padmanabhan N, Howell A, Rubens RD: Mechanisms of action of adjuvant chemotherapy in early breast cancer. Lancet 1986 (ii):411-414

10 Brickner H, Mouridsen HT, Rank F et al: Evidence of a castration-mediated effect of adjuvant chemotherapy (CT) in a randomized trial of cyclophosphamide mono-therapy versus CMF in premenopausal stage II breast cancer. Proc Am Soc Clin Oncol 1985 (4):56

11 Valagussa P, Bonadonna G: Mechanism of action of adjuvant chemotherapy in early breast cancer. Lancet 1986 (ii):1035-1036

12 Ludwig Breast Cancer Study Group: Combination adjuvant chemotherapy for node-positive breast cancer: inadequacy of a single perioperative cycle. N Engl J Med 1988 (319):677-683

13 Ludwig Breast Cancer Study Group: Prolonged disease-free survival after one course of perioperative adjuvant chemotherapy for node-negative breast cancer. N Engl J Med 1989 (320):491-496

14 Anderson JR, Cain KC, Gelber RD: Analysis of survival by tumor response. J Clin Oncol 1989 (1):710-719

15 Kaplan EL, Meier P: Nonparametric estimation from incomplete observation. J Am Statist Assoc 1958 (53):457-481

16 Peto R, Pike MC, Armitage P et al: Design and analysis of randomized clinical trials requiring prolonged observation of each patient. Br J Cancer 1977 (35):1-39

17 Cox DR: Regression models and life tables (with discussion). J R Stat Soc B (Methodology) 1972 (34):187-220

18 Fisher B, Costantino J, Redmond C: A randomized clinical trial evaluating tamoxifen in the treatment of patients with node-negative breast cancer who have estrogen-receptor-positive tumors. N Engl J Med 1989 (320):479-484

19 Kaufmann M, Jonat W, Caffier H, Kreienberg R, Hilfrich J, Abel U, Maass H, Kubli F: Adjuvant systemic risk adapted cytotoxic +/- tamoxifen therapy in women with node-positive breast cancer. In Salmon SE (ed) Adjuvant Therapy of Cancer. V. Grune & Stratton, Orlando 1987 pp 337-346

# Alternative Methods for Describing Treatment Benefit Including Quality-of-Life Considerations

R.D. Gelber [1] and A. Goldhirsch [2]

1 Harvard Medical School, Harvard School of Public Health and Dana-Farber Cancer Institute, Boston, MA, U.S.A.
2 Division of Oncology, Ospedale San Giovanni, Bellinzona, and Ospedale Civico, Lugano, Switzerland

Breast cancer is a major public health problem; it is estimated that about 200,000 women a year in Europe will be diagnosed with this disease. Ninety percent of these patients have operable disease, i.e., after removal of the primary tumour and the ipsilateral axilla the patient is rendered free of macroscopic disease and thus is potentially cured. More than 60% of these patients are estimated, however, to die of metastatic breast cancer. From a statistical and practical point of view, this fact already defines some limitations on the potential gains that can be achieved by treatments. Specifically, an estimated 40% of women diagnosed with operable breast cancer will die from causes other than this malignant disease. Furthermore, relapses and deaths due to breast cancer in a population occur gradually over long periods of time from diagnosis. In contrast, other malignant diseases such as acute leukaemia or high-grade lymphomas have a much shorter natural history with a high rate of events occurring within weeks or months. This makes the identification of effective therapies an easier task than it is for operable breast cancer. If we focus attention upon the high risk population of breast cancer patients (i.e., those with several involved axillary nodes), we may be unable to identify treatments with curative potential. In fact, because the vast majority of high-risk patients may already have "advanced" subclinical metastatic disease, it is possible that no treatment available today can be curative for these patients.

Unfortunately, the effect of adjuvant systemic therapy in breast cancer has been of modest magnitude. This is demonstrated by data derived from the recently conducted meta-analysis (overview) of all randomised trials investigating adjuvant systemic therapy with either tamoxifen or chemotherapy [1]. The estimates are based upon more than 16,000 women included in tamoxifen trials, and more than 13,000 women included in chemotherapy studies. Despite the statistical significance of the treatment effects identified in these analyses, some have argued that the magnitude of the effects is too small to be clinically significant, especially if one considers the costs of adjuvant therapy, both economic and in terms of adverse toxic effects. Thus, given the real but modest benefits from adjuvant therapies for breast cancer, issues of quality of life as well as quantity of life must be considered.

In this chapter we will explore alternative methods for describing benefits of adjuvant therapies for patients with operable breast cancer. Our goal is to provide clinically useful measures which accurately describe the gains for the entire population of treated patients. A central element of our approach is the aspect of time as a descriptive measure of benefit. Both the duration of time gained by using adjuvant therapy and the quality of this time are important issues for patient-care decision making.

**Table 1.** Magnitude of adjuvant treatment effects in early breast cancer estimated by the overview analysis and expressed as Percent Relative Reduction and as Percent Absolute Reduction of relapses and deaths

| | % Relative Reduction | | % Absolute Reduction | |
|---|---|---|---|---|
| Groups of patients and treatment | Odds of death | Odds of relapse | Estimated mortality at 5 years | Estimated relapse at 5 years |
| *Premenopausal (<50 yrs)* | | | | |
| All chemotherapy | 22 ± 6* | 36 ± 5 | 5.7 ± 1.7 | 12.8 ± 2.0 |
| CMF-containing | 37 ± 9 | 48 ± 7 | 9.3 ± 2.6 | 17.3 ± 3.0 |
| Tamoxifen (all) | -1 ± 8 | 16 ± 6 | 0.8 ± 1.9 | 4.5 ± 2.2 |
| Tamoxifen (≥2 yrs) | 1 ± 9 | 18 ± 6 | 1.7 ± 2.2 | 5.0 ± 2.4 |
| *Postmenopausal (≥50 yrs)* | | | | |
| All chemotherapy | 4 ± 5 | 19 ± 4 | 0.8 ± 1.4 | 6.7 ± 1.7 |
| CMF-containing | 9 ± 9 | 25 ± 7 | 1.9 ± 2.1 | 7.4 ± 2.5 |
| Tamoxifen (all) | 20 ± 3 | 33 ± 3 | 5.7 ± 1.0 | 11.4 ± 1.1 |
| Tamoxifen (≥ 2 yrs) | 23 ± 4 | 38 ± 3 | 6.1 ± 1.1 | 12.8 ± 1.3 |

* Percent reduction ± standard error

Data from Early Breast Cancer Trialists' Collaborative Group [1], and the Long Report of the Collaboration

## Estimating the Magnitude of Treatment Effects

Several measures are used to describe treatment effect differences. Table 1 shows results from the overview [1], referring to the magnitude of the treatment effects in 2 different ways. The *percent relative reduction* emphasises the decrease of avoidable events within 5 years, ignoring the population of patients who would not have an event even if not receiving the treatment. The *percent absolute reduction* focuses on the difference in the percent of patients who would not have the event within 5 years if treated, compared with the control population. If the major endpoint of interest is to determine if treatment reduces the risk of relapse or death, then exclusively the percentage relative reduction in odds of relapse and death is to be considered. In this case, the chance for remaining alive and free of disease even with no treatment is completely ignored; the overtreatment for a proportion of the patients is not an issue. This point of view represents a type of "insurance mentality" which focuses entirely upon the risk of an event and ignores the costs in case no event occurs.

Looking at the subpopulations which have the largest magnitude of treatment effects in Table 1 (i.e., CMF-treated premenopausal patients and tamoxifen-treated (≥ 2 yrs) postmenopausal women), the contrast between the relative and absolute reduction in deaths or relapses is striking. The almost 50% relative reduction in the odds of relapse translates to a less than 20% absolute reduction for CMF-treated premenopausal women. Similarly, an almost 25% relative reduction in the odds of death for the postmenopausal women treated for 2 or more years with tamoxifen, translates into a 6% absolute reduction in estimated 5-year mortality.

The apparently small magnitude of absolute reduction in odds of deaths for the 2 populations mentioned above (9.3% and 6.1%, respectively) leads some to express concerns about overtreatment. It is argued that 90.7% of the CMF-treated patients and 93.9% of the tamoxifen-treated patients are "overtreated", having either died despite treatment or remained alive even if untreated. These estimates, however, consider the situation only at one point in time. Claiming that 90.7% of premenopausal women are "overtreated" by CMF ignores completely those patients who benefited in terms of increased survival prior to 5 years and also those who are destined to benefit beyond 5 years. Thus, a more comprehensive estimate of treatment effect is provided by the relative reduction of avoid-

**Table 2.** Baseline prognosis at 5 years. Overall survival (OS) percent and disease-free survival (DFS) percent of "controls"

| | OS % | DFS % |
|---|---|---|
| *Premenopausal (<50 yrs)* | | |
| All chemotherapy | 66.2% | 47.9% |
| CMF-containing | 63.6% | 42.7% |
| Tamoxifen (all) | 71.3% | 53.3% |
| Tamoxifen (≥ 2 yrs) | 71.0% | 54.0% |
| *Postmenopausal (≥50 yrs)* | | |
| All chemotherapy | 66.2% | 47.1% |
| CMF-containing | 65.0% | 45.3% |
| Tamoxifen (all) | 67.7% | 51.8% |
| Tamoxifen (≥2 yrs) | 70.5% | 53.6% |

Data from Early Breast Cancer Trialists' Collaborative Group [1], and the Long Report of the Collaboration

able events. In order to use the relative reduction measure for clinical decision making, however, the additional aspect of baseline risk for the population must be considered. The fact that a treatment is effective at reducing events need not automatically require that it be used for an entire population of patients. The baseline prognosis of patients treated in control groups within the overview of randomised trials on adjuvant chemotherapy and tamoxifen illustrates the issue. Table 2 shows the 5-year baseline prognosis in terms of overall survival and disease-free survival by age and by type of treatment analysed in the overview [1]. Within 5 years, about 40% of the patients who entered trials of CMF chemotherapy were estimated to remain disease free if not treated with this combination. Thus, almost 60% had the potential to benefit from CMF as of the 5-year time point. The tamoxifen trials included patients with a better baseline prognosis: in fact, the 5-year estimated disease-free survival percentage was 54%. Patients will continue to relapse and die from breast cancer as follow-up extends beyond 5 years. It is important to recognise, therefore, that the proportion of patients who might benefit increases with longer follow-up. Thus, while the relative reduction in avoidable events is the preferred measure to define treatment effect, baseline prognosis over time is required to identify costs of treatment. It is, therefore, clear that, in order to approach the definition of net gains of treatment for a given population from a patient-care decision-making point of view, data about the relative magnitude of effect, the baseline prognosis of the population over time, and, an issue discussed later in this chapter, the burden of toxic effects of the treatment, must all be considered.

The baseline prognosis is different for various populations of patients and some factors

**Table 3.** Estimated 5-year OS% and DFS% according to nodal status, oestrogen receptor (ER) status and trials (Numbers of patients are shown in parentheses)

| | Tamoxifen trials | | Chemotherapy trials | |
|---|---|---|---|---|
| | OS % (16,513) | DFS % (15,541) | OS % (9,069) | DFS % (8,172) |
| **Nodal status** | | | | |
| NO | 86 | 75 | 84 | 75 |
| N- | 83 | 74 | 83 | 72 |
| N1-3 | 78 | 64 | 78 | 63 |
| N4+ | 56 | 38 | 55 | 38 |
| N+/unknown | 64 | 49 | 59 | 41 |
| ER++ | 78 | 65 | - | - |
| ER+ | 76 | 65 | - | - |
| ER- | 61 | 54 | - | - |
| ER unknown | 70 | 54 | - | - |

Data from Early Breast Cancer Trialists' Collaborative Group [1], and the Long Report of the Collaboration

**Table 4.** Issues related to evaluation of magnitude of treatment effects in a premenopausal patient population based on data provided by the overview and by common medical practice

| | CMF-containing trials 5-year % | | | Tamoxifen ≥ 2 years 5-year % | | |
|---|---|---|---|---|---|---|
| | Baseline DFS % | Relative reduction in odds | Absolute reduction in % relapse | Baseline DFS % | Relative reduction in odds | Absolute reduction in % relapse |
| Overview derived: | 42.7 % | 48 ± 7 | 17.3 ± 3.0 | 54% | 18 ± 6 | 5.0 ± 2.4 |
| Medical issues: | Treatment with significant burden of subjective toxic side effects | | | Treatment with little or no side effects | | |
| Hypothetical "low-risk" population: | 80% | 48 | 8.5 | 80% | 18 | 3.0 |

which influence prognosis have been defined. Data on 2 of these factors were also available from the overview [1] and relate to nodal status (including number of axillary nodes involved) and oestrogen receptor (ER) content in the primary tumours. Table 3 shows the estimated 5-year overall survival (OS) percentage and disease-free survival (DFS) percentage according to nodal status and oestrogen receptor status for the tamoxifen and chemotherapy trials. The data provide information for all treatment groups and age groups and represent an intermediate estimate between the control cohorts and the treatment cohorts within the trials. These estimates give the possibility to quantify how much is potentially gainable in terms of avoided relapse or death (within the 5-year time frame) for the different risk groups. The node-negative (N- and N0) subpopulations have an estimated mortality percentage at 5 years of slightly more than 15%. The chance of relapse by this time for the entire overviewed node-negative population exceeds 25% and is probably even more than 30% if therapies which provide modest benefit are not used. These results are significantly higher than previously reported relapse rates which did not exceed 20% at 5 years [2-4].

Table 4 shows the information which one uses for extrapolating the data and preparing them for an indirect comparison of treatment options. For a young patient population (< 50 years old) which was entered to CMF adjuvant chemotherapy trials, the absolute reduction in the percent of patients who relapse is estimated as 17.3%. Assuming that the relative reduction in the odds of relapse is 48% also in a population of patients with a rather low recurrence rate (e.g., node-negative, oestrogen receptor-positive patients), for which an estimated baseline DFS at 5 years is 80%, the absolute estimated reduction in relapses is 8.5%. Similarly, for the trials which investigate adjuvant tamoxifen therapy for more than 2 years of treatment, the absolute gain for the younger age cohort decreases from 5% to 3%. The absolute gains are used in an indirect comparison of relapse reduction achieved by different treatment modalities. Specifically, for the population having an 80% 5-year DFS, the 48% reduction in odds of relapse from chemotherapy and the 18% reduction in odds of relapse from tamoxifen provide absolute reductions of 8.5% and 3.0%, respectively. These absolute differences are considered by many to be similar enough to indicate that the less toxic treatment (or in fact no adjuvant treatment at all) should be used for this "low-risk" patient population. The possibility that the 10-year disease-free survival, even for the low-risk population, might be 70%, and that the 20-year figure might be as low as 50%, is not considered by those who rely upon the 5-year time point as a basis for defining potential maximum therapeutic gain.

## The Relevance of Time for the Individual Patient

Information regarding treatment benefit is based upon observations made for a patient population. This must be translated into terms which are relevant for the understanding and the care of individual patients. While reductions in odds of death or relapse are understandable to economists, insurance salesmen and a few epidemiologists [5], the way common mortals intend gains of treatment relates to increased survival time (either free of relapse or overall). Recently, Kim et al. [6] reported that patients preferred to obtain information on symptoms of disease recurrence, progress of illness and duration of treatment, while the physicians emphasised prognosis as being the most important information to communicate, an opinion not shared by the patients. This might be a reflection of the difficulty in describing prognosis in terms of duration of freedom of disease or survival time rather than percent free of disease and alive at a given time.

An attempt to translate prognosis into time measures for an individual patient has been made by using mean or median times observed from a population. Similarly, a common way of expressing treatment effect is to use the difference in terms of median times. The median is the amount of time reached (either alive or free of disease) by 50% of the patients in a given population. Recently, Henderson et al. [7] summarised the results from one of the oldest clinical trials of adjuvant chemotherapy [8] to describe treatment effects in 2 different ways: Figure 1 describes the 10-year survival results observed for premenopausal, node-positive patients in the first Milan CMF study. Figure 1A indicates the absolute differences between survival curves calculating the vertical differences between the curves at 3, 5 and 10 years. Figure 1B indicates the estimation of survival time gained by a given percentile of the population. As mentioned before, a usual measure is to compare the median survival times to present a treatment difference in terms of time. In this example, however, which is representative for studies of operable breast cancer, the median for the treatment group has not yet been reached (i.e., the time at which 50% of the CMF-treated patients are estimated to remain alive is beyond 10 years). The surrogate percentile used to obtain a difference between the control group and the treated group has been taken to be 60%, and the time gain has been observed as 3.5 years. This provides some clue to a time gain which might be understandable for patients who wish to be informed on this issue. Some may interpret this presentation of the data as indicating that the treatment might lead for some patients to an increase in survival of 3.5 years or

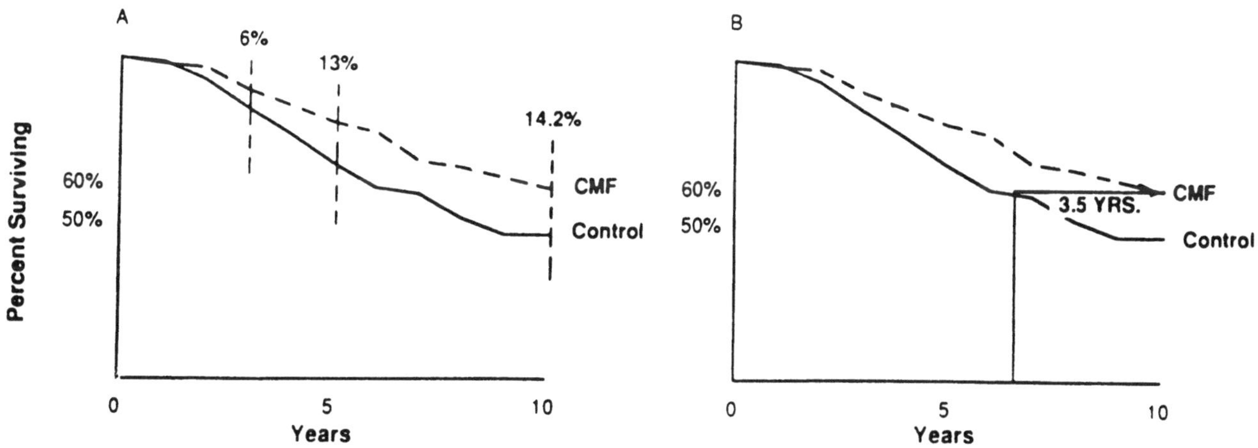


**Fig. 1.** Overall survival (OS) comparison for premenopausal patients treated in the Milan CMF trial. A) Vertical differences between the OS curves at 3, 5 and 10 years after study entry. B) Difference in survival time at the 60th percentile is shown (because median survival has not been reached by 10 years for the treated group). Reproduced with permission from Henderson et al. [7], p 1232

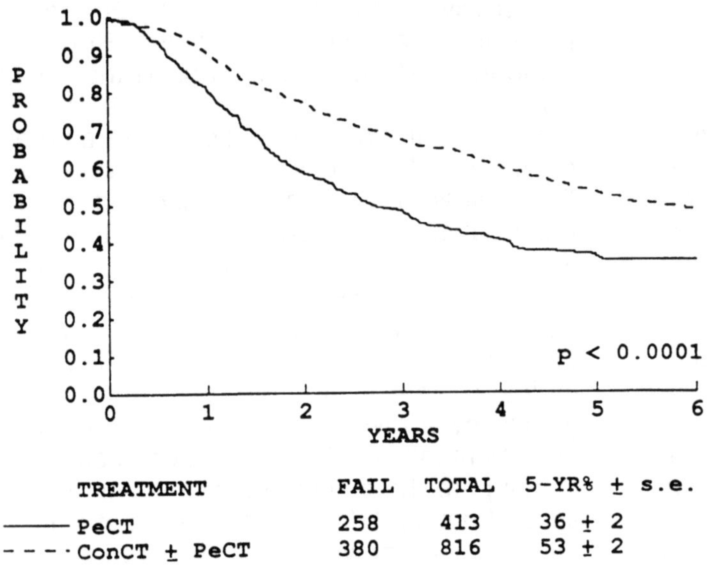


**Fig. 2.** Disease-free survival for 1229 node-positive breast cancer patients treated with one cycle (days 1 and 8) of perioperative chemotherapy (PeCT) versus 6 months of conventionally-timed chemotherapy with or without the perioperative cycle (ConCT ± PeCT)

more, and that this difference is statistically significant. It is clear, however, that if one chooses a different percentile, varying amounts of time gained would be reported. For example, at the 30th percentile no difference between the groups can be represented within 10 years because this patient percentile remains alive whether treated or not. If one takes the 75th percentile (the time at which 75% of the patients are still alive), the difference between the CMF-treated group and the control group is about 2 years. Clearly, the expression of time gained depends upon which percentile of the population is considered. Furthermore, the differences between times might be stretched if the slope of the survival curves is relatively flat at the percentile chosen to define the treatment differences. Thus, for describing treatment benefit for adjuvant therapy of operable breast cancer in terms of *time gained*, alternative methods are required.

One approach is to consider the differences in average amounts of time obtained for patients in the treated group of a clinical trial compared with the control group. This is represented by the area between the survival curves. Figure 2 describes the disease-free survival curve for 1229 patients with N+ breast cancer entered in trial V of the International Breast Cancer Study Group (formerly Ludwig Trial V). In this trial [9], 816 patients were treated with a prolonged chemotherapy (6 or 7 cycles of CMF combination = ConCT ± PeCT) and 413 patients received a short course of perioperative chemotherapy (= PeCT). The results at 4 years' median follow-up time show a significant advantage in terms of DFS (Fig. 2) which appeared early during follow-up. Table 5 describes the DFS percentages and differences between the 2 treatment groups by year (Table 5A).

An alternative description of the treatment differences is illustrated in Table 5B. The area under the disease-free survival curve is calcu-

**Table 5.** Trial V, N+ disease-free survival (5-year median)

**A Differences expressed as DFS percents:**

| Year | ConCT ± PeCT | PeCT | Difference |
|---|---|---|---|
| 1 | 90% | 80% | + 10% |
| 2 | 76% | 58% | + 18% |
| 3 | 67% | 48% | + 19% |
| 4 | 60% | 40% | + 20% |
| 5 | 53% | 36% | + 17% |

**B Differences expressed as average DFS months:**

| Year (months) | ConCT ± PeCT (months) | PeCT (months) | Difference (months) |
|---|---|---|---|
| 1 (12) | 11.6 | 11.1 | + 0.5 |
| 2 (24) | 21.5 | 19.3 | + 2.2 |
| 3 (36) | 30.1 | 25.6 | + 4.5 |
| 4 (48) | 37.7 | 30.8 | + 6.9 |
| 5 (60) | 44.5 | 35.4 | + 9.1 |

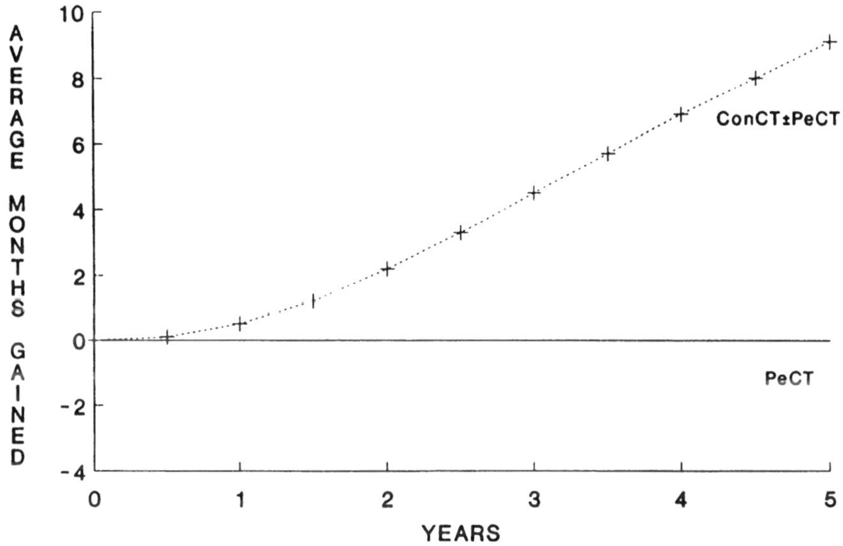


**Fig. 3.** Average months of disease-free survival time gained by ConCT ± PeCT compared with PeCT as a function of time from study entry

lated for each treatment up to the year being evaluated. The result, called the restricted mean [10], represents an estimate of the average amount of time that patients remain free of relapse for the 2 treatments. For example, within 12 months patients who receive 6 or 7 months of adjuvant treatment (ConCT ± PeCT) remain disease free for an average of 11.4 months compared with 10.8 months for patients who receive one cycle of chemotherapy (PeCT), an average gain of 0.6 months for the ConCT-treated population to this time point. By 5 years (60 months), the average gain for the longer duration treatment has increased to 9.1 months. The increasing amount of average time gained is shown graphically in Figure 3. This represents an option for describing the evolution of the average gains in DFS over time which, as an average value, is relevant for the entire population of treated patients. This overcomes the obstacle encountered with the method illustrated in Figure 1, in which the time reported as gained (3.5 years) applies only for a specific arbitrary percentile.

The average DFS gained is represented by the area between the DFS curves for the 2 treatment groups up to 5 years. By considering the individual percentiles of the populations from the top to the bottom of the vertical axis of the DFS plot (Fig. 2) (shortest DFS to longest DFS), we can describe the component parts of the average gains. This is similar to the horizontal calculation of time at an arbitrary percentile that was illustrated in Figure 1, but accounts for the time gained by *all* percentiles of the patient population. Figure 4 shows the percentile gain function (or quantile distance function [11]), indicating the disease-free survival time gained within 5 years by the patients who receive prolonged chemotherapy compared with those who had a single cycle of treatment, according to population percentile. The percentile plot indicates the gains for patients with the shortest DFS time on the left and for those with the longest DFS time on the right. The vertical amounts are those obtained by considering the horizontal distances between PeCT and ConCT curves in Figure 2 at each percentile with a vertical boundary at 5 years. The results of this analysis indicate a secure gain for a proportion of patients (47%), a potential continuing gain for 17%, and a lack of gain for some of the patients (36%) who did not relapse but were not expected to do so because their virtual controls remain disease free. The 53rd percentile is the "maximum gainer" (3 years of DFS gain) at 5 years and represents the selected gain displayed in Figure 1 for the CMF series.

## Quality-of-Life Considerations

The description of treatment benefits for patients with operable breast cancer traditionally has relied upon evaluation of survival times and time free from disease recurrence. A major component of the cost of treatment -

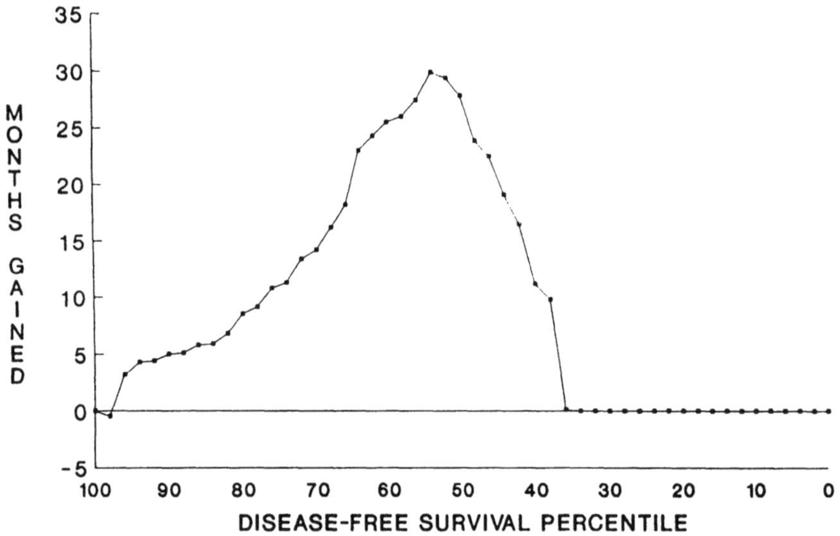


**Fig. 4.** Quantile distance function based on comparing the disease-free survival curves for ConCT ± PeCT minus PeCT within 5 years from study entry. The months gained are calculated as the horizontal differences between the DFS curves (Fig. 2) for each percentile of the patient population. Percentiles on the left had the shortest DFS times, while those on the right had the longest times for both groups

toxic effects of adjuvant systemic therapies - was only considered separately. The integration of the impacts of side effects of drugs upon life quality and the influence of the therapy upon disease-related symptoms were partially ignored due to the methodological difficulties to include all these components in a single evaluation.

Methods to incorporate quality-of-life considerations into the main analysis of clinical trial comparisons were described in previous issues of this European School of Oncology Monograph [12,13]. These involve the development of new endpoints as follows:

1. TWiST: Time Without Symptoms (of disease) and Toxicity (of treatment) with the definition of
   a) TOX: survival time *with* subjective toxic effects of treatment,
   b) REL: survival time following symptomatic relapse,
   c) TWiST: survival time with TOX and REL *completely* subtracted.

**Table 6.** Average months of Q-TWiST accumulated during time from randomisation. Different values of the utility coefficients are illustrated

| | Months from randomisation | | | | |
|---|---|---|---|---|---|
| | 12 | 24 | 36 | 48 | 60 |
| **Q-TWIST** ($u_t = u_r = 0.5$) | | | | | |
| ConCT ± PeCT | 9 | 20 | 30 | 38 | 47 |
| PeCT | 11 | 21 | 30 | 38 | 44 |
| **OS** ($u_t = u_r = 1$) | | | | | |
| ConCT ± PeCT | 12 | 23 | 34 | 43 | 52 |
| PeCT | 12 | 23 | 33 | 42 | 50 |
| **SDFS** ($u_t = 1$; $u_r = 0$) | | | | | |
| ConCT ± PeCT | 12 | 22 | 31 | 39 | 47 |
| PeCT | 11 | 20 | 28 | 34 | 39 |
| **TWIST** ($u_t = u_r = 0$) | | | | | |
| ConCT ± PeCT | 6 | 16 | 25 | 33 | 41 |
| PeCT | 11 | 20 | 27 | 33 | 38 |

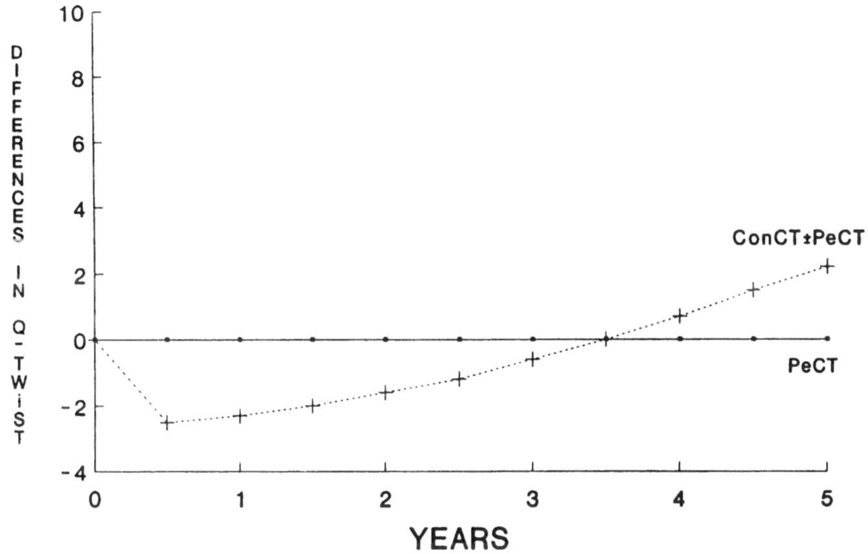


**Fig. 5.** Average months of Q-TWiST ($u_t = u_r = .5$) gained by ConCT ± PeCT compared with PeCT as a function of time from study entry

2. Q-TWiST: The incorporation of quality-adjusted survival time to allocate *some value* to life periods with toxicity and relapse. $U_t$ and $u_r$ represent utility coefficients taking values between 0 and 1 to reflect the worth of TOX and REL relative to TWiST.

$$\text{Q-TWiST} = \text{TWiST} + u_t \times \text{TOX} + u_r \times \text{REL}$$

For comparative evaluation of treatments in randomised trials, the methodology provides a measure for assessing survival times of a *useful* quality (i.e., including times with toxicity and with symptoms as *costs* in the description of the overall "economy" of the treatment programme). Applying the method to the 1229 N+ patients in International Breast Cancer Trial V, and considering $u_t = u_r = 0.5$ (i.e., life with toxic effects and with symptomatic relapse is "worth" half of life without toxicity and relapse), values per year of average Q-TWiST are obtained (Table 6). In addition, average values of overall survival (OS), disease-free survival (DFS) and TWiST are shown. Figure 5 displays the evolution of the differences in average values of Q-TWiST ($u_t = u_r = 0.5$) over time, comparing the prolonged duration of chemotherapy (6 or 7 cycles) with the single short course of chemotherapy given to the control group. This graphical presentation illustrates the early "deficit" in average Q-TWiST for the ConCT group due to early toxic effects of longer duration experienced by *all* patients. A delayed benefit is due mainly to the significant reduction in symptomatic relapse. In fact, the ConCT group starts to gain Q-TWiST at 2 years compared with controls. At 5 years, the net gain is on the average 6 months for the ConCT versus PeCT, despite the early burden of subjective toxic effects.

At 5 years, a Quantile-Quantile analysis [14], similar to that shown in Figure 4 describing DFS differences, can also be applied incorporating the TOX and REL data for quality-of-life oriented comparison. Figure 6 shows this analysis applied to the Q-TWiST data from Trial V. In this case, the percentile gain function identifies a portion of the patient population receiving ConCT which has a net loss Q-TWiST relative to their corresponding percentiles of PeCT "controls". The comparison with Figure 4 illustrates the difference between the DFS gains at 5 years and the Q-TWiST gains at the same time point of follow-up. Portions of the prolonged treatment group that have a "net loss" in Q-TWiST are evident, while the overall average assessment favours ConCT, and some patient percentiles experience substantial gains in quality of life.

**Fig. 6.** Quantile distance function based on comparing the Q-TWiST ($u_t = u_r = .5$) distributions for ConCT ± PeCT minus PeCT within 5 years from study entry. The months gained are calculated as the horizontal difference between the Q-TWiST distributions for each percentile of the patient population. Percentiles on the left had the shortest Q-TWiST, while those on the right had the longest Q-TWiST for both groups. Patient percentiles which lost Q-TWiST in ConCT relative to PeCT are on the left due to early relapse in the ConCT group, and on the right due to no relapse in PeCT "controls"

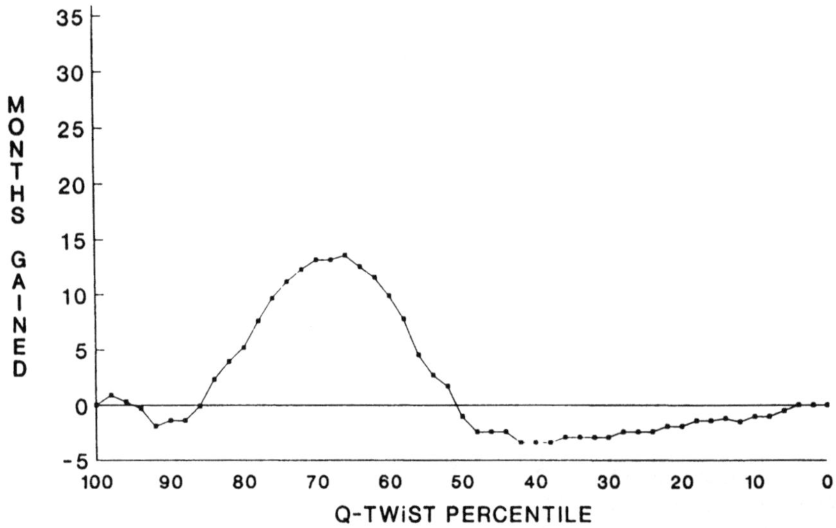


## Conclusions

Statistical methods for treatment comparisons are designed to distinguish real effects from the observed differences that are subject to the play of chance. The alternative methods discussed in this chapter are intended to provide summary measures to describe the magnitude of treatment effects. The usual measures refer to portions of the patient population and emphasise either the avoidable events (relative reduction) or the consideration of the entire population at some point in time (absolute reduction describing survival). Time gained by treatment is an appealing approach from a patient-care point of view. Integration of "life-with-events" and "life-with-toxicity" into those descriptive methods offer a tool for communicating costs and benefits of adjuvant therapies for breast cancer.

## Acknowledgement

We thank the patients, physicians, nurses, and data managers who participate in the International Breast Cancer Study Group trials. We also gratefully acknowledge the support for central coordination, data management and statistics provided by the Swiss Cancer League, Cancer League of Ticino, Swiss Group for Clinical Cancer Research, Australia-New Zealand Breast Cancer Study Group, and Frontier Science and Technology Research Foundation.

## REFERENCES


1 Early Breast Cancer Trialists' Collaborative Group: Effects of adjuvant tamoxifen and of cytotoxic therapy on mortality in early breast cancer. An overview of 61 randomized trials among 28,896 women. N Engl J Med 1988 (319):1681-1692

2 Fisher B, Slack NH, Katrych D et al: Ten-year follow-up results of patients with carcinoma of the breast in a cooperative clinical trial evaluating surgical adjuvant chemotherapy. Surg Gynecol Obstet 1975 (140):528-534

3 Nemoto T, Vana J, Bedwani RN et al: Management and survival of female breast cancer: Results of a national survey by the American College of Surgeons. Cancer 1980 (45):2917-2924

4 Valagussa P, Bonadonna G, Veronesi U: Patterns of relapse and survival following radical mastectomy. Cancer 1978 (41):1170-1178

5 Amir M: Considerations guiding physicians when informing cancer patients. Soc Sci Med 1987 (24):741-748

6 Kim CJ, Park JW, Youn JS et al: A study comparing the perception of patients, nurses, and doctors about the educational needs of cancer patients. Taehan-Kanho 1989 (28):53-66

7 Henderson IC, Harris JR, Kinne DW, Hellman S: Cancer of the breast. In: DeVita Jr VT, Hellman S, Rosenberg SA (eds) Cancer. Principles and Practice of Oncology. JB Lippencott, Philadelphia 1989 pp 1197-1268

8 Bonadonna G, Valagussa P, Rossi A et al: Ten-year experience with CMF-based adjuvant chemotherapy in resectable breast cancer. Breast Cancer Res Treat 1985 (5):95-115

9 The Ludwig Breast Cancer Study Group: Combination adjuvant chemotherapy for node-positive breast cancer: inadequacy of a single perioperative cycle. N Engl J Med 1988 (319):677-683

10 Kaplan EL, Meier P: Nonparametric estimation from incomplete observations. J Amer Statist Assoc 1958 (53):457-481

11 Laake P, Laake K, Aaberge R: On the problem of measuring the distance between distribution functions: analysis of hospitalization versus mortality. Biometrics 1985 (41):515-523

12 Gelber RD, Goldhirsch A: Evaluating the benefits of therapies for breast cancer. In: Cavalli F (ed) Endocrine Therapy of Breast Cancer II. European School of Oncology Monograph. Springer Verlag, Berlin 1987 pp 20-32

13 Gelber RD, Goldhirsch A, Simes RJ, Glasziou P, Castiglione M: Integration of quality-of-life issues into clinical trials of breast cancer. In: Cavalli F (ed) Endocrine Therapy of Breast Cancer III. European School of Oncology Monograph. Springer Verlag, Berlin 1989 pp 27-36

14 Gelber RD, Gelman RS, Goldhirsch A: A quality-of-life-oriented endpoint for comparing therapies. Biometrics 1989 (45):781-795

FSC
www.fsc.org
MIX
Papier aus verantwortungsvollen Quellen
Paper from responsible sources
FSC® C105338

If you have any concerns about our products,
you can contact us on
**ProductSafety@springernature.com**

In case Publisher is established outside the EU,
the EU authorized representative is:
**Springer Nature Customer Service Center GmbH**
**Europaplatz 3, 69115 Heidelberg, Germany**

Printed by Libri Plureos GmbH
in Hamburg, Germany